# Nightmares

# NIGHTMARES

## How to Make Sense of Your Darkest Dreams

Alex Lukeman, Ph.D.

M. EVANS

*Lanham • New York • Boulder • Toronto • Plymouth, UK*

M Evans
An imprint of Rowman & Littlefield
4501 Forbes Boulevard, Suite 200
Lanham, Maryland 20706
www.rowman.com

**Library of Congress Cataloging-in-Publication Data**

Lukeman, Alex, 1941–
    Nightmares : how to make sense of your darkest dreams / Alex
Lukeman.
        p.   cm.
    Includes index.
    ISBN 978-1-59077-236-2
    1. Nightmares.  2. Dream interpretation.  I. Title
BF1099.N53 L85 2000
154.6'32—dc21                                            00-037134

Distributed by NATIONAL BOOK NETWORK

Book design by Teresa Steadman and Rik Lain Schell

Printed in the United States of America

*To everyone who has struggled with the fear
brought on by dark and difficult dreams.*

# CONTENTS

# ACKNOWLEDGMENTS

First and foremost I want to acknowledge the dreamers who shared their nightmares with me and provided the raw material for this book. It's not easy to talk about nightmares for most people. I hope their stories will help others deal with their own dark dreams.

Although I will never have the privilege of studying with them, two great masters deserve credit for the inspiration and guidance they have provided for me through their pioneering spirit and seminal works on dreams and the mysteries of the unconscious psyche: Sigmund Freud and Carl Gustav Jung. These men opened the door to the study of dreaming as a serious topic for understanding the human soul.

As always, I am grateful to W. Brugh Joy, M.D. It was Brugh who first cleared the way for me to reach a genuine understanding of dreams.

Finally I want to thank Noah and Gayle for their unflagging support and advice.

# INTRODUCTION

Are you one of the millions of people around the world who have terrifying and disturbing dreams? For most of us, nightmares are the kinds of dreams we easily remember but would rather forget. I've been working with dreams of all kinds for over twenty years. In my private practice as a psychotherapist, and when I am conducting groups and workshops, people frequently tell me about terrifying and difficult dreams.

I became interested in nightmares and other kinds of dreams because I've always been a vivid and active dreamer. It always seemed to me that dreams were too complex to dismiss as simply meaningless and random neural firings of an overactive brain. My intuitive feelings have been born out by years of studying dreams and observing their relevance to our daily lives.

I've learned nightmares can be an important resource for self-knowledge and spiritual and emotional discovery. Many times I've seen the discussion of a nightmare lead to a solution for some deeply troubling problem or personal difficulty. Frightening dreams are particularly significant, because no one gets a nightmare until there is a real need for attention by the dreamer.

This book offers a way of understanding nightmares that has worked for me and for many others. I wrote it because I wanted to create a practical guide for dealing with nightmares, a map anyone might follow through the shadow land of dark and frightening dreams. The techniques and suggestions are tested and proven through years of practical application. If you have nightmares, you can follow the suggestions given and get relief and results.

Lots of things can lead to having a nightmare. You will find plenty of information within these pages to help you determine the cause. Whatever it may be, the good news is that you can do something about it by paying attention and making an effort to understand the underlying message of the dream. Then, perhaps, you won't need to have the nightmare again.

All of the nightmares used in this book are in the original words of the dreamers. More than half the examples given are from women. About seventy-five percent of the people who work with me are women, and in general women tend to participate in the groups and workshops I conduct about dreams more frequently than men. The interesting thing is that nightmares have no respect for gender and couldn't care less about the sex of the dreamer. Since all nightmares use the context of the dreamer's life as a basis for the symbolic images seen in the dream, men's and women's dreams reflect the gender experiences of waking life. But both sexes dream of all the themes presented in these pages.

Please use this book as a resource, a friendly guide for self-discovery. Good luck on the journey!

*Alex Lukeman*
*Fort Collins, Colorado*

# HOW TO USE THIS BOOK

Everything in these pages is designed with one goal in mind—to help you make sense of your nightmares and make whatever choices needed to eliminate them. There are three parts to the book, plus a helpful glossary of common nightmare symbols located at the end and an index to make it easy for you to find specific subjects within the text.

Part One will show you how to look at dreams in general and nightmares specifically. It may not turn you into an instant expert, but it does offer practical information about the dream language of nightmares and how to understand it. If you have always wondered why people dream and have nightmares, you will find some answers in this section. Part One also contains a "nightmare quiz" that's fun to take and can reveal a lot about what might be causing your nightmares. Your answers provide clues about whatever it is in your life situation that might be contributing to your disturbing dreams. Once you know what is at the root of your nightmares, you can take steps to do something about it. Knowledge is power when it comes to dark dreams.

Part Two is a series of chapters focusing on different nightmare themes and scenarios that are universal in nature. These kinds of nightmares appear to people all over the world, regardless of ethnic or cultural background. The images of your dreams may be unique, but the themes are not. You are not alone. Open to a chapter containing nightmares with a theme similar to your own and you will find something to help your particular situation. It will be general (because it's not *your* dream) but each chapter gives practical information about the same theme and underlying dynamic as the one in your nightmare.

Sometimes just by seeing that others have had the same awful experience you can begin to put the dream in proper perspective and get a handle on the upset. You don't have to be an expert on interpreting dreams to gain understanding and relief. Read through the dreams of others and see if what the dream meant for them applies in some way to you. Working with many people over the years I've had good luck with this approach. You can get good results too.

If you don't find the specific theme of your nightmare listed in the table of contents, then take a look at chapter 17 in Part Two. You might find it there.

Part Three moves to a more general look at nightmares. Here you will find material on Post Traumatic Stress Disorder (PTSD) nightmares, nightmares that warn us of potential or actual physical health problems, children's nightmares and teen nightmares. Each chapter presents useful, down-to-earth ideas and suggestions.

Use the suggestions as practical guidelines. For example, if you are ill or are concerned about your health, the health chapter presents several kinds of dreams foreshadowing or commenting on illness and helps you understand how to tell the difference between a regular nightmare and one that may have immediate health considerations.

If you have kids or teens in your home who have bad dreams, you may find something here to help you make life a little easier. Children's nightmares and teen nightmares are similar to the nightmares of adults, because they contain fearful scenes meant to convey something from the unconscious to conscious awareness. The focus and images of the dreams may be different (because they are not adults), but the same principles for understanding apply.

If you want to know how to get control of your nightmares or how to deal with them after you wake up, go to the last chapter. Here you will find proven suggestions for taking the fear out of nightmares, including an ancient technique called conscious or lucid dreaming.

At the end of the book is a glossary of common nightmare symbols with possible meanings and thoughts that can help point the way to what the symbols of your nightmare mean for you. Use this to get an idea of how the meaning might apply to your own situation.

All in all, there is quite a lot of information about dealing with nightmares scattered throughout the book. Generally speaking, you will find practical tips and suggestions located near the end of each chapter as well as throughout the text. Look for the bulleted or highlighted lists and use the information wherever it seems right for you. Most of all, enjoy yourself and know that you can get a handle on your darkest dreams.

# PART ONE

---

# Nightmare Basics

# 1

## WHAT ARE NIGHTMARES?

You are standing on an unfamiliar shore, looking out over a dark and threatening ocean. The light is strange and flat overhead—a sense of foreboding and approaching disaster fills you with dread. Behind you lies a strange city on a hill, filled with people who are all starting to look nervously toward the horizon. Suddenly an enormous wave appears in the distance. It rushes toward you, towering higher and higher until it fills the sky above you. You want to run away, but you can't get your feet to move quickly in the sand—your legs feel heavy and useless. The wave is almost upon you, blotting out the light as you struggle to lift your legs. The roar of the water fills your ears, people are screaming and running all around you, and you can see the furious, churning water at the curling edge of the wave as it begins to break far, far above. You feel completely helpless before the raging, overwhelming power of the wave. You know you are about to die and fear turns your blood cold. You scream—and wake sitting bolt upright in bed.

You've just had a nightmare. Welcome to the ranks of millions who wake up on any given night in terror, their minds filled with horrifying visions of death and destruction, hearts pounding, the taste of fear in their mouth—normal people just like you.

Dreams often disappear like a wisp of smoke with the daylight, but not nightmares. Unlike other dreams, nightmares have such an impact upon our waking mind that we usually remember them. If you have nightmares, read on—in these pages you will find understanding and help.

The important thing to understand about nightmares is that they serve us in some way. Nightmares aren't bad in and of themselves—they may be disturbing to us, but once we understand how to work with them, they can be a valuable and practical resource. They give us information we can use in our waking life. Nightmares warn us that we are caught up in some internal conflict needing resolution for the sake of our well-being. Stress and trauma, fears and insecurities, feelings of inadequacy, pressures of work, relationship problems, life challenges and physical health can all trigger a nightmare. Most people wish they never had that dark dream. But think of it another way. Wouldn't you rather have warning when something was wrong? All nightmares are dreams, but fortunately for our peace of mind all dreams are not nightmares. The only difference between regular dreams and nightmares is in content. It is the frightening or deeply disturbing emotional component that sets the true nightmare apart.

## Why We Dream

If you ask a dozen different psychologists or sleep experts why we dream you're likely to get a dozen different answers. There are two popular and completely opposite points of view about why we dream. The scientific and physiological approach favored by professional sleep researchers and many psychologists takes the position that dreams don't have any meaning at all. For most scientists dreams are nothing more than random neurological events, which may or may not be related to learning and memory functions.

The scientific approach requires hard evidence that can be objectively studied. About the only kinds of dream evidence sci-

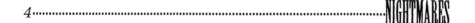

entists can pin down are recordings of brain waves from sleeping subjects. REM (Rapid Eye Movement) states of consciousness, in which dreams usually occur, can be observed and recorded on scientific equipment, but no one has yet managed to capture an actual dream for objective study. From this point of view, dreams are seen as internal processing of life events by our brain and are not thought to have any intrinsic meaning.

On the other end of the spectrum are those who think dreams are in fact full of meaning and that the meaning can be understood. Dismissed as "believers" by the scientists, these people see dreams as important communications from within, providing valuable and practical information for living. You can count me with these folks. I am definitely a believer, and I base my beliefs on years of practical experience and observed results. I'm not alone: from ancient physicians like Hippocrates to modern giants like Freud and Jung, many have taken the position that dreams are actually openings onto a landscape of the soul, revealing expanded possibilities of self and spirit. Nightmares sound a wake-up call to rmind up of those possibilities.

## Some Thoughts about Dreams

Sometimes people think an external event like watching a horror movie will produce a bad dream. If that were true, then the dream might not have much meaning—it would simply be a kind of nightmarish replay of the film, with you in one of the starring roles! But my experience is that this isn't what happens. The dreaming mind picks up on the movie images and gives them to you in a dream because they get the desired symbolic message across. From my point of view there are no accidental or meaningless images in a dream. They all have personal meaning—some more than others—and it is a mistake to dismiss them as simply the result of something occurring during the waking day.

We dream because we must, for physiological reasons and because dreams tell us things we need to know about ourselves. Health, relationships, work issues and difficult problems of all kinds are addressed in our dreams. Dreams are critical to health. When someone is deprived of dreams they begin to hallucinate; if dream-deprivation is carried far enough, death can result. Throughout history, dreams have encompassed everything from prophecy and revelation to the discovery of benzene and insulin.

Most of us don't really want to take the time to learn how to interpret our dreams—and who can blame us? Learning to understand dreams is like learning a foreign language: it takes desire, time and a willingness to learn. The language of our dreams is symbolic and the symbols are both universal and personal. It can be confusing to try to sort out the different possibilities and levels of meaning a dream may contain. But when it comes to nightmares, we usually don't need convincing that it's worth our trouble to understand.

In many tribal cultures throughout the world, nightmares are seen as a bad omen. A member of the tribe who had a nightmare on the eve of a great hunt or an important ritual might not be allowed to go with the rest. His dream would keep him apart from the others. He might even have to go through a purification ceremony before he could return to his usual place in the society. Dreams of the dead can be seen as particularly bad news; it is thought that the dead person is actually returning. Since this is against the natural order of things, such a dream may be viewed with great alarm. A nightmare is a bad omen if your culture or belief system says it is.

## Why We Have Nightmares

The nightmare is a way for our unconscious mind to get our conscious, waking attention. There are many reasons why we can have a nightmare. Scientists are right when they say dreams help our minds process the events of our daily lives; every day we attempt to integrate enormous amounts of information and experience. Sometimes those events are difficult to take in. The stress of modern living creates fertile ground for the appearance of a nightmare. The trend toward depersonalization in the workplace, the pressures of family and relationships, the failings of our society and

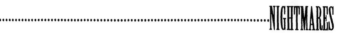

the highly visible horrors that appear on nightly television all contribute to the making of a true nightmare. Illness, medications, stress, trauma and impossible workloads play their role in the creation of "bad dreams." We are all potential candidates for the nightmare experience, simply because of the random and often difficult nature of our lives.

Nightmares caused by psychological distress can occur because of current events or because of something that has happened in the past. For example, people with PTSD (Post Traumatic Stress Disorder—see chapter 19) often report recurring dreams or repetitive nightmares. Combat vets, people who have suffered some horrible event like an airplane crash, victims of crime, people in high-stress occupations like flight controllers or policemen—all of these folks can have bad nightmares from time to time, sometimes every night. In these cases, the nightmare is a response to the experience of unacceptable stress or events. The dreams are trying to help resolve the fear and psychic conflict, with the implication that something needs to be done to change things.

Unfortunately for those of us who lead relatively uneventful lives, it's not necessary to be in one of those specialized, high-risk or high-stress situations to get a nightmare. We may never be victimized by traumatic crime yet dream of rape and violation.

Of course to get any practical use from a nightmare, we must get a good sense of what it means. That requires a look at the basic nature of dream imagery.

## The Language of Dreams and the Nature of Dream Images

The language of dreams is written in symbols—images that carry layers of meaning. We already have a lot of experience understanding symbols, whether we know it or not. For example, why do we send roses to a loved one on Valentine's Day? We might not consciously think about it, but the rose has long been a symbol of romantic love. The red can represent passion and the dedication of the heart, the green of the leaves symbolizes life, and the thorns of the stem remind us that love is not always as smooth and pain-less as we might like. There are other meanings for the rose as well: if a rose appears in your dream, you can be sure it's more than just another pretty flower.

Understanding dreams of any kind begins with feeling into the layers of meaning connected to the dream symbol. Dream imagery can roughly be divided into two very broad categories: imagery born out of our personal experience of life and imagery that arises from an impersonal store of symbolic image and meaning common to all humankind. Dreams often combine the two, in an effort to get across the message we need to hear.

This is an important concept for true understanding. No one has a problem seeing symbols as personal, but the idea that we may be tuned in through dreams to something universal in nature can get a lot of people shaking their heads and rolling their eyes. In this category we come across prophetic dreams, dreams that sometimes change the course of human events. It's an idea at least as old as the biblical story told in Genesis of Joseph and Pharaoh. Do you know the story?

## *Joseph and Pharaoh*

The short version: Joseph is sold into slavery by his jealous broth-ers. Falsely accused by Potiphar's wife of sexual advances, he ends up in one of Pharaoh's prisons. While there he interprets two dreams for two prisoners. Both interpretations are borne out by events that come to pass. One prisoner, Pharaoh's royal baker, is executed. The other prisoner, the royal wine-bearer, is set free as Joseph predicted. Years later Pharaoh has a nightmare. He dreams of seven lean cows eating seven large ones, then of seven lean ears of corn eating seven full ones. Pharaoh wakes distraught, unable to get help from the best necromancers in Egypt.

The wine-bearer remembers Joseph's ability with dreams and tells Pharaoh, who summons Joseph from prison. Joseph tells him the dreams predict a time of famine coming to Egypt, seven lean years after seven good ones. Pharaoh puts Joseph in charge of preparing for the disaster. Now in a position of great power, Joseph saves Egypt from starvation and is reunited with his family.

Because Joseph was able to truly interpret a dream, the most powerful ruler in the world set Egypt on a fourteen-year journey of preparation. For seven years the people were taxed and grain stored in huge silos. In the next seven years of terrible drought Egypt was saved, while the rest of the region suffered terribly. I wonder what would happen if the leaders of today's world paid more attention to their dreams?

Joseph and Pharaoh were responding to something possessed of wisdom that appeared in dreams, something mysteriously beyond their personal selves. In the Bible this wisdom and guidance was attributed to God. In the language of modern psychology one way to describe it was coined by Carl Jung, a Swiss doctor who developed the branch of psychotherapy called Analytical Psychology. He called it the "collective unconscious." Whatever it is or whatever you call it, it is real and can be experienced in dreams. The trick is to learn to tap into the wisdom.

## Universal Themes and Symbols

There are universal themes and symbols occurring in nightmares, regardless of culture, time or place. They appear in dreams to all humans and transcend situation and cultural experience. We can understand something about our nightmares if we can understand something about the themes and symbols that occur for all of us. The table of contents for this book reflects many of these themes. As you read further you will find many examples of symbols, both universal and personal.

Anyone who watches television or goes to the movies has been exposed countless times to many frightening symbols and themes of human experience. Good movies (even many bad ones) use powerful symbolic cues to convey feeling and intensity, engaging the audience in a virtual experience of the story being told on the screen. The most successful movies tap directly into our sub-conscious minds, without the need for outer, rational evaluation. The images of the film go right past the filters of our outer mind and produce an instant, non-rational response.

Take *Psycho*, for instance, the well-known Hitchcock horror film. The most famous scene in this movie, a classic in its own right, is the shower scene where someone—we don't know who—murders the character played by Janet Leigh with a large kitchen knife. Viewing the film we are instantly caught by the intensity of the attack. Conscious knowledge of watching a movie is frozen by a perception the murder is real. We respond on a visceral and unthinking level, because the scene speaks to a universal fear we all carry—the fear such a thing could happen to *us*.

In dreams we seem to have a real experience. We don't usually know we are dreaming—it appears real, just as in a movie scene. The very successful series of films beginning with *Nightmare on Elm Street* exploits our common experience of dreams as real, building horrific events and truly nightmarish sequences on the themes and symbols filling our worst nightmares. The horror movies of our culture reflect back to us an underlying psychic pool of fearsome images that is a dark part of our human heritage. Like nightmares, they trigger our psychic alarms.

## *Getting to the Meaning*

Fortunately it's possible to grasp the meaning of a nightmare and thus put an end to the need for having it. Even though your nightmare holds a particular meaning uniquely yours, by looking at dreams similar to yours you may get an understanding of what your dream means for you. This is true even if you are no "expert" on dream interpretation. The chapters in this book dealing with specific themes can help you do that. You can find relief.

It does help to keep a few basic guidelines in mind. It's impossible to define any given dream symbol appearing in a nightmare, like a poisonous snake or a relentless stalker, in a way always correct for everyone. Your dream is a specific, personal dream. The trick is to get to the meaning the dream symbol has for you. How do you do that?

## *Seven Keys for Finding Relief from Nightmares*

The points below provide a strong foundation for effectively dealing with your nightmares. Let's consider each one in turn.

**1. REALIZE THE NIGHTMARE DIDN'T OCCUR JUST TO SCARE YOU,
BUT HAS MEANING AND PURPOSE. THIS IS ABSOLUTELY FUNDAMEN-
TAL TO LOOKING AT NIGHTMARES.**

Sometimes people think when they have a nightmare they are
being victimized by their own dreaming mind. Nightmares are so
disturbing that there is a strong tendency to push them out of our
thoughts as quickly as possible. That's not always easy.

Nightmares occur for specific reasons. The reason may be physical, such as serious illness or as an effect of medication; in that
case the meaning of the dream may bear directly on the physical
problem. The reason may be psychological; then the dream is trying to point out some underlying psychic context rooted in the
past or the present, definitely relevant to a current life situation.

Whatever the reason, it is important enough so that our dreaming mind decides a nightmare is needed. That's all it can do—it
can't make us interpret the significance and act accordingly. That's
up to us. Once we understand the dream communication we learn
something we need to know about ourselves, practical information
directly affecting our well-being.

**2. YOU HAVE AN INNATE ABILITY TO UNDERSTAND AND GAIN
RELIEF FROM THE DREAM.**

When you discover the meaning of a dream, relief appears. The
nightmare may indicate something you need to do, some action to
take, some possibility to explore—you would not have the dream
unless something within you thought you could make sense of it.
Something in you brought you the dream—actually "dreamed it
up." That same something knows the meaning of the dream and
will be happy to help you understand it.

**3. DON'T BE AFRAID TO LOOK AT HORRIFYING IMAGES, OR THINK THAT BAD IMAGES MEAN BAD THINGS ABOUT YOU.**

People are often shocked by what appears in their nightmares. This is a good place to point out that the unconscious mind, the source of our nightmares, doesn't seem to care about things we normally hold to be important. Morality, ethics, civilized rules of behavior, cultural mores and taboos—all of these mean nothing to the unconscious. It is a mark of human evolution that we have created civilized societies in which we can live and work together without acting out the primal urges forming the basis of our ancestral heritage.

Dreaming about actions utterly repugnant to our waking mind does not mean there is something bad or wrong about us. It only means we are being asked to take notice of the symbolic acts of our dreams as a way of understanding something. Don't be afraid to think about the nightmare. There is a reason and a purpose why you dreamed it. Try to set aside your natural judgments and fears and see the dream objectively for what it is—a dance of images created from within that grabbed your awareness through its power and horror. Your challenge is to make sense of the dream, not dismiss it out of hand.

**4. LEARN TO STEP AWAY AND CONSIDER THE IMAGE OBJECTIVELY, WITHOUT EMOTION, IF POSSIBLE.**

It's not easy to understand something when we are caught up in an emotional response. If we simply react to the dream, we won't understand anything. We have to set aside our feelings and see the nightmare images for what they are—symbols containing meaning for us.

Here are a few tips for viewing the dream objectively:

- Pretend you are watching a movie or television show—you are not actively engaged, just observing the story and drawing conclusions about the characters and action.
- Take a few deep breaths, then tell the story out loud to yourself (or a sympathetic listener). Do this three times, and you

will find that the emotional charge has been greatly reduced. This works!

- Remind yourself as much as you need to that it's a dream, even though it felt so real. Just a dream, but important because it is trying to tell you something.
- Get a paper and crayons and draw the images as best you can— create a picture of the dream. This can help you realize the meaning and defuse the emotional charge.
- In your mind's eye, visualize yourself in a peaceful setting. Examine each of the scenes in the dream, always returning to the sense of peacefulness and calm with which you started.
- Relax!

The secret to emotional discharge is found in familiarity and in an effort to look at the problem with as much awareness as you can muster. Face it squarely and it will diminish in its power.

**5. IF YOU GET AN IDEA OF THE MEANING, YOU GET TWO GOOD RESULTS: YOU WON'T HAVE TO HAVE THE DREAM AGAIN AND YOU HAVE PRACTICAL ADVICE FOR YOUR REAL, OUTER LIFE.**
Sometimes just making an effort to understand alleviates the need for another nightmare, or for the same one to return. When we really get the meaning of a dream, it is a visceral feeling—we feel the correctness in our body. Such a dream always has practical implications for waking life. If you can't see the connection, it only means you have to look harder to find it.

For example, suppose you realize overwork and exhaustion provoked the nightmare. The implication of the dream is to do something to relax, reduce stress and take care of yourself. Once you grasp the meaning of a nightmare you will not need to have it again—unless you ignore the message, in which case it may come back stronger and more intense than before.

**6. REMIND YOURSELF THAT NIGHTMARES CAN OPEN THE DOOR TO LOVE AND HEALING IN BOTH A PSYCHOLOGICAL AND A PHYSICAL SENSE. THEY ARE A GIFT FROM YOUR UNCONSCIOUS MIND, EVEN**

**THOUGH THEY SEEM FRIGHTENING WHEN THEY OCCUR.**

It may seem odd to think of a nightmare as a gift, but that is what it truly is. It helps to think in this way. By discovering the meaning of a dream it's possible to release old hurts, heal old emotional wounds or burdens or detect illness that may be dangerous. You may trigger a potential within you for broader understanding and appreciation of your life. That's in addition to just finding relief from the dream because you got a handle on it! You would not have the dream unless it was so important your sense of well-being and inner peace depended on it. I'd call that a gift, wouldn't you?

**7. LET YOUR MIND RELAX; FREELY ASSOCIATE IMAGES, FEELINGS AND MEMORIES.**

The man who rediscovered the importance of dreams in modern times was Sigmund Freud. He encouraged his patients to express a free-flowing association of thoughts and images, which he then used as a basis for therapy. You don't have to be a psychoanalyst to do the same. The secret to finding the meaning of your nightmares lies in opening yourself to a relaxed flow of imagery and thoughts, allowing ideas and memories to surface until something triggers a sense of correctness about the meaning.

For example, suppose you dream of standing naked in front of a large crowd, unprepared to deliver a speech. This is a common dream, a nightmare for many. What could this mean? Let your mind roam over the images of the dream. Standing naked = no clothes = embarrassed = exposed = vulnerable. You are feeling exposed and vulnerable about something. You have to deliver a speech, but you are unprepared. Speech = communication. Unprepared = without needed information or knowledge or practice = inadequate to the task. If you combine feeling vulnerable and exposed with an inability to communicate based on feeling inadequate to the task, you are getting a sense of the meaning. Then when you look at your waking life you will find some situation that mirrors the concern in the dream. Perhaps there's a big presentation coming up at work or there's a need to prove yourself in some way that others will notice. Now you know why you had the nightmare and can do something to better prepare yourself or calm your fears. This is how free association works. Look at each important piece of the dream and then think about the underlying associations. It takes practice, but you can learn to do it.

## The Nature of the Unconscious Mind

As I'm writing this chapter I feel the need to say more about the unconscious mind and the way it communicates with us through all dreams, especially nightmares. This book is not meant to be a psychological and academic look at nightmares; it's meant to be a practical guide. Yet it is impossible to talk about nightmares with any real depth and not use terms like "unconscious." It's also impossible to interpret dreams fully without honestly questioning ourselves about what they might mean. Sometimes that honesty leads us to places we'd rather not see and to questions we would rather not ask.

The unconscious mind isn't like our waking mind. Our waking mind has learned many things about how it is supposed to be in the world. Depending on what it is we have learned, what culture we come from and a host of other life factors, we become the kind of person we are. We think of ourselves as being a certain way—not in detail, but with an overall sense of self. For example, we learn that it is not all right to just take what we want when we want it. If we refuse to learn that lesson we may end up in prison, because society has mechanisms in place to protect the majority from the predators among us.

The unconscious mind, however, does not play by the same rules. In the unconscious the predator is alive and well, along with a large cast of other interesting and sometimes not very nice characters and personas that cannot be safely expressed in their primal form. The conscious mind becomes the arbiter, imposing restrictions, rules, and context. But the unconscious will have its say regardless of our efforts to regulate it. This can lead to some difficult inner conflicts and stressful responses in waking life. Those conflicts show up in nightmares.

You don't have to have a degree in psychology to understand dreams, but you do have to have compassion for yourself and a genuine desire to seek out the meaning. The unconscious mind is unexplored territory for most and no maps are available. There is no science of understanding dreams and nightmares, no perfect lab procedure that can always produce a satisfactory and repeated result. When it comes to dreams, we are all travelers together on a road into the unknown, marked only by the fleeting, ephemeral images of our dreaming minds.

Simply because nightmares are so disturbing, they often refer to things we don't want to know about, hidden corners of our being we have managed to avoid bringing into the light. Sometimes the dream challenges deeply held convictions or beliefs. Usually when that happens we will reject the message. More frequently, we simply don't understand it. That is a way to protect our ideas about ourselves, a way to avoid making waves in our lives. I don't know anybody who wants waves made in their life. We all tend to go into powerful denial if confronted with a potential wave-maker.

Here's a true story to illustrate what I'm talking about. Some years ago I was acting as a strategic business consultant, applying what I know about how people think and act to the corporate world. I always tried to bring a dose of common sense into the meeting room. For example, do you think it might be a good idea to ask production line employees if they have any ideas about improving productivity when productivity is declining? Sounds logical, doesn't it?

My partner and I were making a modest proposal to the executive team of a well-known major American corporation. When we brought up the idea of surveying employees on the production line for suggestions and ideas, the chief executive of the company said, "But what if we find out something we don't want to know? We might have to do something about it!" I couldn't believe he had actually said that. Scary, isn't it? Here was the highly paid CEO of a big-time company refusing to consider anything that might force him to change his ideas about how it all should be done. Needless to say we did not land the job.

Our minds can be just like that business executive when it comes to understanding and acting upon the content of our nightmares. We don't want to hear about it. We go into denial and shut down the possibilities. It may be a common response but it's not a good way to do business.

When you have a nightmare and try to make sense of it, you may not like what you discover. After all, the dream wasn't any fun and disturbed you, so why would you necessarily like the information it was trying to give you? If you were ill, you might not like a medical treatment that saves your life, either, but when alternatives are considered the choice is made to go ahead. Don't be like the president of that big firm. Take in the information, then use your common sense and trust in yourself to make the adjustments the dream is calling for. You will never regret it if you do.

## The Shadow

The realm of the unconscious is vast compared to what we are aware of in our outer minds. It is like the ocean, infinite and deep—one reason the ocean often represents the unconscious in dreams. Unconscious material is hidden from outer awareness. What usually comes up in nightmares is disturbing and concealed negative psychic content—we can't see it without specific training and are mostly unaware it is there. Carl Jung called this psychic content "the Shadow." This is why I think of nightmares as "dark" dreams. They are born of the darkness within us and carry the shadow content into the light of our waking consciousness.

Are you familiar with *The Shadow* of radio fame? That famous show of the past featured a hero who learned "the power to cloud men's minds" in the mysterious Orient. I loved listening to this show when I was a boy. Lamont Cranston (the hero) could confuse and confound the bad guys by asserting his shadow powers. We unwittingly do the same to ourselves—we confuse and confound ourselves by hiding important self-knowledge in the shadow of the unconscious mind.

Shadow content is difficult for our outer minds to accept. That's why it is hidden in darkness. It takes a particular kind of temperament to actively seek out and discover shadow material, and it is definitely not a journey for most of us. There is a problem though—we may not choose to explore those darker reaches but our unconscious doesn't much care whether we want to or not. If something in us thinks we need to take a look at something unpleasant, all it has to do is give us a nightmare. This is another reason we have disturbing dreams from time to time.

This book is not a psychological exploration of how to understand the shadow, but it is a very practical exploration of shadow material. All nightmares are by definition conceived in the shadow. My interest here is not in revealing the nature of the shadow but in helping you get practical results that are observable in your waking life. I want to help you find relief from dreams that send chills down your spine. If you follow the suggestions given and allow yourself to relax and feel into the ideas about different nightmare themes, you will get good results. Let's begin with a quiz to help you understand what might be causing your nightmares.

# 2

-- -- -- -- -- -- -- -- -- -- -- -- -- -- -- -- -- -- -- --

# A NIGHTMARE QUIZ

Nightmares are an inner story we tell ourselves. A nightmare lets us know we are feeling out of control and unsafe in our lives, stressed or disturbed about something. The way to deal with disturbing dreams is to identify the nature of the problem and make changes to alter the situation. How can we do that?

The first step is to find out what is bothering you. Sometimes that can be difficult. For example, if the cause of your nightmares is rooted somewhere back in your childhood, it might take some effort to understand it. The good news is that it's in the here and now where resolution can take place.

Quite often the cause of a nightmare is found in the present, in a current life situation. When that is the case, once you know what the problem is you can choose to do something about it—then you won't need to have the dream.

Here is a simple Nightmare Quiz you can take to help identify possible reasons for having a nightmare. Once you understand the reason, you can take steps to change your situation.

Each beginning statement in the quiz is followed by four choices that best describe how you feel. No one answer is better than any other—in other words, this is not a quiz to see how many answers you can get right. At the end of the quiz I'll tell you how to interpret the results, and from there we can get a quick snapshot of what might be causing your bad dream. Statements 8 and 9 are gender specific; answer only the one that applies to you, not both! Statements 11 and 12 address relationships; answer only the one that applies to you. Grab your pencil, and have fun with it.

## *Nightmare Quiz*

**1. My work situation is:**
   a. just great—no problems at all
   b. pretty good, but I work too hard
   c. not so good—I wish I could get something better
   d. awful—anything would be better than this

**2. In general, my relationships are:**
   a. lots of fun and very satisfying
   b. good—not many problems, and I get along well with most people
   c. not so hot—people don't seem to see me for who I am
   d. miserable—I wish people would treat me better

**3. In my childhood I was:**
   a. loved and nurtured as much as I needed
   b. taken care of pretty well—my parents did the best they could
   c. disciplined a lot and told that I was wrong a lot
   d. abused (sexual, verbal, psychological, physical)

**4. In my life I generally feel:**
   a. in charge, safe and secure, good about my life
   b. pretty much on top of things and heading where I want to go
   c. stressed and worried a lot about things—money, family, work and more

    d. unable to get what I want and not in control—I'm scared and angry about what might happen

**5. I think that people are:**
    a. mostly good, basically trustworthy
    b. likeable, but you do need to be careful
    c. mostly out for what they can get for themselves
    d. dangerous and untrustworthy

**6. The world is:**
    a. a great place to live, and it's a great time to be alive
    b. really interesting, but you need to watch your step
    c. a very dangerous place, but I am careful and stick to familiar ground
    d. hell on earth

**7. Our society is:**
    a. the best there is and doing great—we're on the right track
    b. good, but there are a lot of problems
    c. in serious trouble, and I think about it a lot
    d. falling apart, and we'd better learn how to protect ourselves

**8. (For women) In general, I think men are:**
    a. great—hey, what would we do without them?
    b. doing the best they can, but they sure need some work
    c. pretty dense—men don't understand much and I'm careful around them
    d. dangerous—you can't trust them at all

**9. (For men) In general, I think women are:**
    a. great—thank God we've got women
    b. good to have around—whatever the problems, I'm glad they're here
    c. pretty dense—I wish we didn't have to put up with them
    d. out to get you—you can't trust them at all

**10. I think that horror movies are:**
    a. good fun—you can't take that stuff seriously
    b. entertaining—if it's a good one, I'll go see it
    c. disturbing—I usually avoid them
    d. awful—I won't see one and I don't understand why anyone would

**11. I'm single. In general, my relationships are:**
   a. really great
   b. pretty good—I feel there's someone out there I can relate to
   c. not so hot—everybody seems to want something from me
   d. lousy—I feel very alone

**12. I'm married. In general, my relationship is:**
   a. wonderful
   b. good—marriage has been worth it
   c. not very good—I wish it was a lot better
   d. terrible—I feel trapped and angry, sad and frustrated

**13. My life so far has been:**
   a. very smooth and working out the way it should
   b. challenging, but things usually work out OK
   c. uncertain and insecure—I've had a lot of troubles
   d. terrible—you wouldn't believe all the bad things I've seen and experienced

**14. I feel most secure:**
   a. all the time—it doesn't matter when or where
   b. when I know what's going on and have choice about what I'm doing
   c. when I'm home and don't have to be out there dealing with people
   d. when I'm totally in control and know I can defend myself in any way needed

**15. In my work I feel that:**
   a. my work is satisfying and useful—I can make it the way I want
   b. I mostly like what I do
   c. my job is boring and doesn't really mean much
   d. my job is something I hate, but I have to do it

**16. When I was growing up, my family was:**
   a. very supportive and loving
   b. supportive, but I wish they had shown more love to me
   c. difficult to live with and I never quite knew what to do to please them
   d. abusive—I couldn't wait to get out of there

**17. The way I deal with strong emotions is:**
  a. by embracing them—I allow myself to feel them and talk about them
  b. cautiously—I'm not too comfortable with them, but I try to express them
  c. reluctantly—I don't feel comfortable at all with strong emotions
  d. by avoiding them—I don't let myself feel such things

**18. The best way to be in life is:**
  a. to do your best to take care of things and have a good time
  b. to take it day by day and figure it will all work out
  c. to watch your step—it's risky and dangerous
  d. to remember that life is a jungle—you've got to get what you can because someone else might get it first

**19. When I go to bed at night I usually expect that:**
  a. I'll get a restful night's sleep and have pleasant dreams
  b. I'll probably get enough sleep and may remember some dreams
  c. I'll toss around and finally go to sleep, but I won't feel rested in the morning
  d. I'll lie awake and I won't like the dreams I have when I finally get to sleep

**20. I have nightmares:**
  a. never—I can't even recall ever having one
  b. very infrequently, but I do get them sometimes
  c. once or more a month
  d. almost every night

**21. In general, I would rate my stress levels as:**
  a. very low
  b. average, but I don't think it's much of a problem
  c. high—I'd like to be more relaxed
  d. very high—I'm stressed all the time

**22. My personal health is:**
  a. very good—I feel healthy and vital
  b. pretty good—there's nothing to worry about
  c. not so good—I take medications and I feel unhealthy much of the time
  d. poor—I'm very worried about it

**23. The kind of work I do is:**
   a. relaxing and pleasant, most of the time
   b. a job—it could be a lot worse
   c. difficult and stressful
   d. dangerous and high-pressured

**24. When I feel stressed out, I:**
   a. take a few days off and relax
   b. make some time for myself and try to relax more
   c. get irritable and frustrated—I don't know what to do about it
   d. feel as if I'm going to explode, so I stuff it and keep going

**25. The idea that all of us have unconscious thoughts about life is:**
   a. very familiar to me
   b. seems reasonable to me
   c. an idea I don't know anything about
   d. complete hogwash—it's just psycho-babble

**26. Dreams are:**
   a. interesting windows opening onto our inner selves
   b. part of sleeping and often entertaining
   c. disturbing and strange
   d. just random garbage from the mind—why pay attention to them?

**27. My beliefs about spiritual things are:**
   a. very important to me—they guide my life
   b. important, but I don't think about it much, except when I worship
   c. not very important—I'm not sure there's anything to it
   d. that it's all just superstition

This is just a pop quiz in a book about nightmares—don't take it too seriously. Some of the statements might get you thinking about something you'd rather not think about, but that may be exactly why you are having nightmares: something needs to be thought about that isn't high on your list of favorites.

Here's how to score: give yourself a 4 for every (a) response, a 3 for every (b) response, a 2 for every (c) response, and a 1 for every (d) response, then total your score. Since statements 8, 9, 11 and 12 are directed at two different groups of people, the highest possible score is 100 (25 answered questions × 4 = 100). The lowest possible score is 25 (25 × 1 = 25). A score of 100 is very unlikely; a score of 25 is also very unlikely. Almost everyone (including myself) will fall somewhere between these two extremes.

A score of 75 to 100 indicates you don't seem to have much of a problem with nightmares. You are probably reading this book because the subject interests you or someone you know does have nightmares frequently. A score of 60 to 75 indicates that there are several reasons why you might be getting nightmares. These range from job stress to difficulties with childhood experiences or current relationships. A score of 40 to 60 indicates you are under strong emotional stress and are feeling a lot of pressure in different areas of your life. You really need to make some changes, because the level of stress you are carrying is bad for your health and bad for your peace of mind—it's a perfect setup for nightmares. If you scored under 40, I strongly recommend you think about professional counseling to help you get through some of the issues you are facing.

All of the statements can be loosely grouped into broader categories. These are Work, Relationship, Childhood and Family, Stress, Life in General and Dreams. Many of the statements could easily fit into more than one category. Feel free to consider them in any way you like. Responding with (c) or (d) usually indicates higher levels of emotional, mental or physical stress. The exception is with the two statements on dreams. These are an instant snapshot of how you think about dreams and the unconscious part of our awareness that brings dreams (and nightmares) to us.

By looking at the responses you chose in each category, especially where you gave yourself a (c) or (d), you can get an idea of what is behind your darkest dreams. Once you have an idea, you can do whatever might be necessary to change things. There is always some action you can take to shift whatever underlies the creation of your nightmares. Then you won't need them anymore.

## Work

Statements 1, 15, and 23 deal with work. Work is a common source of stress and insecurity in general and nightmares in particular. Work is so unsatisfying for so many that it has become a significant cause of much that goes wrong in our society. Think how often we hear about somebody who "lost it" over a work situation and "went postal." There's a big difference between working hard at something you enjoy and working hard at something you hate because your survival seems to depend upon it. Unfortunately, many of us fall into the latter category.

Unresolved, work-related stress can be a powerful source of nightmares. Work is a daily occurrence for most of us: we spend a large amount of time in our work environment, whatever it may be. You don't have to earn your living in a dangerous place like a steel mill or a police car to feel threatened. Our mind picks up on all the cues of our lives, positive and negative, and incorporates them into our dreams.

Do you dream of being relentlessly chased by dark figures in business suits? Perhaps your job is part of the problem, along with a poor relationship to authority figures telling you what to do. Dreaming of careening down the highway, out of control? Perhaps your nightmare is reflecting feelings of frustration and an inability to direct one of the major areas of your life—your job. Going to war in your dreams, attacking and killing your enemies? The nonsense of your workday may be appearing in your dreams, a kind of psychic safety valve and signpost of increasing levels of frustration.

If the dream setting is like your workplace, take a realistic look at the stress created by your work situation. If it is not balanced by a sense of accomplishment, satisfaction and a feeling that this is right for you, then consider making changes. You can do it, if you plan for it and explore your possibilities for something different. If you don't make the effort, nothing will get better.

People in high-stress jobs with severe and immediate consequences for failure often have nightmares. Police officers, firefighters, emergency medical personnel, military personnel, air-traffic
controllers, miners, heavy equipment operators—the list is seemingly endless. These occupations all include the real risk of serious
consequences, injury and death, either directly or through the
actions of another. If you are in one of these kinds of jobs, then you
are probably highly trained, highly motivated and highly dedicated
to your occupation. You probably aren't going to change anytime
soon. What can you do about nightmares?

The answer is learning how to effectively manage the levels of
stress that go with your job. You may already have heard lots
of helpful suggestions and well-meaning advice. Here's a short list of
suggestions that might help (I apologize in advance if you've heard
them before).

- Take time off to really relax and let go. Get in a hot tub (or a
  hot bath), go for a run, go out for dinner, sleep for a day, go to
  a dumb movie and laugh a lot—whatever you like.
- Lighten up. Laughter is the best, first line of defense against
  stress, and that includes black humor. Black humor is a healthy
  response.
- If something is really getting to you, find a peer who understands and talk about it. If you are comfortable with the idea,
  see a professional who guarantees confidentiality.
- Learn techniques for self-relaxation (biofeedback, meditation,
  visualization, self-hypnosis, breathing—whatever works).
- Learn more about your job—knowledge is protection and gives
  you confidence.
- Remember that you are not the only one who feels the way
  you do.

These tips are very general, but they will help alleviate the job-
related stress you feel. Just beginning to consciously make
changes or apply stress-relieving techniques is often enough to
end a cycle of nightmares.

## *Relationships*

Relationships are right up there with work as a prime cause of nightmares. Not just intimate relationships, although these have enormous impact. All relationships, including the one we have with the rude driver who cuts us off or the waitress at the restaurant where we have lunch can show up in our nightmares. Statements 2, 8, 9, 11 and 12 specifically deal with relationships.

If we don't think people like us or if we think they cannot understand or see us for who we are, we feel isolated and unhappy. This can show up in our nightmares as images of abandonment and loneliness, with no one to hear us or come to our rescue.

If we see members of the opposite sex (or our own!) as threatening and insensitive, men or women in our dreams can take on menacing aspects reflecting our inner insecurities. If we are single and looking for someone to connect with, there is a real possibility of hurt and disappointment. If we are unfortunate enough to be in a bad marriage, we suffer that disappointment every day. Bad relationships can mean it's nightmare time.

Will everyone reading this book who has not had a bad relationship please raise a hand? I can't see you, but I'm willing to bet no one has a hand in the air. Everyone, and I mean everyone, has suffered through a bad relationship. Those past experiences show up in our dreams, reawakened by the things that happen in the present.

Responding with (c) or (d) answers to the statements about relationships simply indicates you may have some real issues regarding men or women and may not find it particularly easy to relate to people in general. You aren't alone, but it can make for a lot of problems that will show up in your dreams. Nightmares caused by poor relationships can be handled by doing something about them. I can't give you a pat solution here—this book is not about fixing relationships, and there are plenty of books already in print on the subject. If you are in an unhappy relationship or have trouble relating to people in a general sense, seek out advice about how to improve your situation. Books, friends, counselors, seminars—there are plenty of resources available for you.

## Childhood and Family

This is a big one. In my private practice I often see people traumatized in some way by the events of their childhood. The problems range from lack of love to severe abuse. Family members can be the most destructive influence of all on a person's life. If you were lucky enough to have a loving and nurturing family, then that's not what is causing your difficult dreams. But if your childhood was an unhappy one, problems rooted in past neglect bear evil fruit years later.

There are only two statements in the quiz referring directly to childhood: 3 and 16. The emphasis is on whether or not you received enough love, in a positive sense, when you were a child. This is an explosive, emotional subject for many people. If you had an abusive childhood and are having nightmares, please think about seeing a counselor. The key to resolution of dark childhood events is found in talking through the experiences and discovering a new level of appreciation and acceptance of self.

One woman I know was sexually abused in her childhood. For years she had a repeating nightmare of desperately trying to climb a slippery rope up a vast, bottomless shaft. She was unable to reach safety, represented by raised ridges on the side of the shaft. In the dream a fall meant certain death. After a time of seeing her counselor the dream changed. Now there were knots in the rope, where she could pause and hold on. Safety wasn't complete, but the situation was definitely better. Those knots represented a growing sense of security and safety within, and the dream was telling her about the progress she was making. She is now happily married and has come to terms with the trauma of her childhood experiences.

## *Stress*

Statements 21 and 24 are specific to stress levels you experience and how you handle them. If you answered (c) or (d) to either of these two, you are a candidate for nightmares. The way we handle stress is critical to our well-being and in our modern society stress has become a national issue. Severe levels of stress affect all aspects of our mental, emotional and physical health. That includes dreams.

If you have been involved in a traumatic incident of some kind, especially if you have been diagnosed with Post Traumatic Stress Disorder (PTSD), you are very likely to have nightmares. These can be flashbacks to the event or a similar dream setting; they can be apparently unrelated, at least as far as the dream imagery goes. PTSD can occur whenever things go really wrong in our lives and we are confronted with our sense of mortality and vulnerability. War, rape, accidents, a death in the family, serious illness, natural disaster, terrorist acts, crimes of any kind against us—these and more can set up a sequence of nightmares, often repeating regularly over a long period of time.

Relief from these kinds of dreams is found in counseling and in letting yourself talk through your feelings and concerns. There are usually support groups of one kind or another available, as well as professionals ready to assist you in every town of moderate or larger size. The nightmares are a normal response to unacceptable levels of fear and stress. For more about nightmares and PTSD, please see chapter 19.

Whatever the source of your high stress levels, please do something to reduce the pressure. There is always something you can do, no matter what the cause. It's a choice. Once you recognize the need, acknowledge it and do whatever is necessary—your peace of mind depends on it.

## Life in General

This is the biggest category of statements in our quiz. Statements 4, 5, 6, 7, 10, 13, 17, 18, 22, 25 and 27 all fall into this category. If you look at the statements, you'll see they focus on issues of control, perception of the world and ourselves, health, our attitude toward other people, our relationship with spiritual ideas and concepts and even how we think about watching horror movies.

It's easy to look at the world or our society and become alarmed about any number of things. What almost all of those things have in common is that they are completely out of our control. We can feel victimized and helpless thinking of terrorism, nuclear threats, incompetent government policies, natural disaster, crime in the streets—all the negative themes that fill our newspapers and television news programs.

When we feel unable to affect events that can have significant and unwanted impact on our lives, we may begin to have disturbing dreams. Now we are dreaming of nuclear war and great floods, or perhaps vicious criminals, dark monsters and evil forces pursuing us down mean dream streets with the intent to kill or maim.

I wish I had a simple answer for the frustrations the greater society and world bring to us. What I do is try to focus on the areas where I can make a personal impact, small as it might be. Since I'm not in a position to tell world leaders what they ought to do (use common sense and be nice to each other, with respect for the differences between us all), I have to find other avenues to balance the frustration I feel about the way things are. If you are having difficult dreams, perhaps you can do the same. Volunteerism is a good solution. Finding a way to help others in your community is great therapy for the troubled mind, and it's free to boot!

During the '70s the cliché about "making a difference" developed. Cliché it may be, but making a difference, even a small one that doesn't shape the destiny of nations or governments, is a way to send nightmares back into oblivion. The reward of "doing the right thing" is very satisfying and nurtures us on many levels. The right thing is always about service to others and helping people when trouble comes, as it usually does sooner or later.

In other words, you are among millions of others if you feel frustrated and sometimes discouraged or angry about the way things are going out there. Let yourself move from criticism to service and you will be amazed at the change it can make in your sleep and dreams.

How you feel about watching horror movies is in this group because the statement reflects something about your ideas and attitudes. I'm not saying you should go watch horror movies! But nightmares so often match or exceed the most horrific offerings Hollywood sends to us, and a desire to avoid anything horrible (like that type of movie) may paradoxically lead to some awful dreams.

Horror movies work because they frighten us with images arising from our collective shadow consciousness. They are nightmares in celluloid (or whatever studios use these days), and the vicarious fear we experience in the theater reminds us uncomfortably of our own vulnerability. Oddly enough, there is real psychic benefit in the vicarious experience. By confronting the scenes in the movie we help ourselves come to terms with our inner demons. It's a process of psychological integration. Denial of the darker aspects of existence is one of the causes of nightmares.

You don't have to go to horror movies. The statement is in the quiz to partially reveal how you think about horrifying images. Do you refuse to allow them into your outer consciousness? That's fine, but you should know they exist anyway within your unconscious; it is part of our human condition—part of our collective shadow. If they begin to show up in your dreams, you need to discover what is provoking them.

Statement 25 is there just to review what you think about the whole idea of humans even having something called the "unconscious." If you think it's all a bunch of hooey, you have lots of company, but you would probably not be reading this book. I am

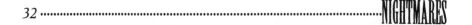

completely convinced, for many reasons, of the reality of the unconscious. You don't have to know much about it and I'm not going to try to explain it in any detail. That would be a book in itself, and in fact there are many serious volumes out there about the subject. All you really need to know is that dreams and nightmares arise from this part of ourselves and appear to us in the language of the unconscious—symbols.

Understanding the unconscious is a task that will never be completed. But we can understand dreams and nightmares by understanding our personal dream language. That takes practice. To make it easier I've included a glossary of some common nightmare symbols at the end of the book. The glossary provides an overview, in a very general sense, of what some symbolic dream language may actually mean. There is also a lot of information in any chapter about specific kinds of dreams. Look up your kind of dream in the relevant chapter and use the similarities to trigger your thinking about what your dream may mean.

Statement 22 addresses health. Poor health is sometimes at the root of disturbing dreams. Prescription medications often affect dream states and brain activity, producing weird and strange dreams. The same is true of alcohol and all of the illegal drugs used for recreation. Illness, fever or infection affects brain activity as well. Serious or terminal illness will show up in dreams, often as a nightmare. It's a natural adjunct, reflecting outer worry and concern and inner awareness that a fight for life is going on.

Years ago I worked with a man who had a massive brain tumor. He was certainly doomed by any reasonable medical standard. Medical tests, including CAT scans, provided a terminal prognosis: he had not long to live. The illness was represented in his dreams as a smoking and shorting television set, a dream metaphor for his damaged brain. However, the dream also included a TV repairman, which seemed to indicate he could survive.

In fact, after some intensive counseling and healing work, he went into a miraculous remission and the tumor disappeared. Then he had another dream, a nightmare in which he realized there was still a monster locked in an underground tunnel behind a closed door. The door was closed, but the monster was waiting behind, ready to leap out and devour him. This dream indicated he had won the battle, but could still lose the war. The monster represented the illness, which had gone into remission but was still present within him. Only time will reveal if the monster can stay imprisoned.

Statement 27 is there to get a quick snapshot of your relationship with spiritual ideas and experience. People with a very strong sense of spirit or who make spiritual teachings important in their lives feel supported and nurtured by their beliefs. It helps them to weather times of crisis and stress, and provides a context of community and support. That, in turn, can reduce the frequency of nightmares.

## *Dreams*

Statements 20 and 26 refer to nightmares and dreams. Responding with (c) or (d) to statement 20 probably explains why you are reading this book. Anyone who has frequent nightmares wants them to go away. The way in which you responded to statement 26 tells you something about your ability to deal with the nightmares you are having. In this case, the (d) response isn't a very good sign, because it means you don't really put any credence behind the idea that nightmares, or dreams of any kind, have significance. If that's the case, there isn't a lot I can say, since this book is based on the premise that nightmares do have significance. From my point of view, relief is found through understanding the dream and taking whatever steps required to effect change.

An (a) response tells you that you are in great shape for the exploration. Most of us will respond with (b) or (c), which are essentially neutral regarding ideas about dreams and the unconscious.

Use the quiz to give yourself a quick profile of how you think and feel regarding the subjects discussed in the sections above. Your responses should give you a rough picture of what problem areas contribute to creating your nightmares.

It's time to start looking at different kinds of nightmares. Ready? Jump in—you won't need to pull the covers over your head.

# PART TWO

---

# Universal Nightmare Themes

3

# INSECTS AND OTHER PESTS

Something bugging you? Maybe you'll have a nightmare about bugs and insects. By now you know that nightmares of any kind are warning us something is up with our inner sense of well-being—something is upsetting our peace of mind. By looking at the specific theme of the nightmare we can get a sense of what is disturbing us. Usually we've ignored the upset—that's why we get the dreams.

Insects and crawly things disturb a lot of people. Insects are very old forms of life. They are good nightmare symbols for basic kinds of problems—problems the mind wants to solve, appearing in dreams as scaly, slimy, crawly, many legged, pincer- and stinger-waving horrible insects.

Insects are usually small, but when there are lots of them they become frightening and can overwhelm almost any defense. Horror movies sometimes use giant insects to instill terror, magnifying our natural aversion into something larger than life. Perhaps you've seen the classic sci-fi movie *Them*, featuring giant mutant ants that attack people and hide in the storm drains of Los

Angeles. Many movies have been made over the years featuring spiders, ants, bees, moths, mantises and other things that fly, crawl, sting and devour.

The other day I was walking in our local shopping mall when I came face to face with a giant praying mantis. I mean a GIANT mantis, ten feet high, a robotic, life-like moving model placed in the mall as part of an educational exhibit for kids. I've got to tell you, the last thing I'd ever want to see is something as big, nasty-looking and ugly as that nightmare creature coming after me. I wouldn't have a chance against it and neither would you unless you had some serious firepower with you.

In our dark dreams insects overwhelm and attack; our primal fears come true.

*I had a nightmare recently. . . . the meaning baffles me. I dreamed pests were overrunning my house. A slew of cockroaches was coming up through a heating vent in the floor. I was panicking, trying to stomp them to death. In my kitchen spiders swarmed out from behind the refrigerator. Rats crawled out from under the stove and I proceeded to grab one around the neck and twist until its neck was broken. I was in a blind panic as I violently killed these creatures, stomping them, squishing them under my feet and breaking their necks. In actuality, it brings tears to my eyes when I have to squish an ant or fly.*

Well, rats aren't technically insects, but the dream still belongs in this chapter. Pests are pests, and that's a key word this dreamer uses to describe the onslaught. Attacked by pests in her kitchen— the setting tells us the bottom line for this dream.

The kitchen is a place where we prepare food. Food = nourishment, sustenance, the stuff of life. This woman is feeling unnurtured, unnourished, beset with many irritating things in her life, attacked from all sides in a place where she should feel comforted. This kind of dream can pop up when there's trouble at home; it can occur because of feeling as if your life is going to hell in a hand basket and that nobody cares about you.

Cockroaches are dirty insects; rats are disease-bearing animals associated with plague, garbage and filth. Spiders are something everybody has an opinion on, but few of us love them. There's an association here with hidden filth, "garbage," something spoiled, something decayed or rotten. OK? Can you see how the association is made?

Even though there is no image of garbage or decay in the dream, by thinking about the nature of the attacking pests we get an idea of what the dream is about. This is the bottom line if you want to understand why you are having nightmares: think about the essential nature of the nightmarish and frightening thing and then let yourself discover the hidden meaning by association.

Whatever is panicking this dreamer in real life is showing up in the dream. What is it that is filthy and spoiled that has to do with nourishing her? I'd put my money on a relationship gone bad— perhaps a cheating husband or betrayal by a friend, business associate, family member or lover. Only she knows.

Here's another buggy dream.

*In my dream I was in bed and it was night. I woke up in my dream, for some reason, and on my floor were bugs. My floor was crawling with worms, scorpions, centipedes and cockroaches. I woke up and looked at the floor, and for the next week I was scared to step on my rug.*

Yech! I'd think about putting my feet on the floor, too, after that dream. The floor is where we stand—our foundation. We say things like, "I felt like the floor dropped out from under me," to convey a sense of losing our foundation, our sense of certainty and security. This dream says the dreamer is feeling very insecure in her life. The insecurity brings out those old primal fears we all keep stuffed inside. In the dream world they look like bugs and worms, crawling everywhere we would put our feet.

Scorpions are interesting dream elements. Scorpions are thought to sting themselves to death. If you are an astrology buff, you know people born under the sign of Scorpio tend to have difficult lives and are often described as self-destructive or self-defeating. Whatever the truth of astrology, scorpions do make an excellent dream symbol for inner judgments and insecurities turned against oneself.

*My dream was that scorpions were entwined and infested in my hair, similar to Medusa and the snakes. I was trying to get them out of my hair by swinging and swatting at them with something in my hand.*

*In reality my hair is cut short like Demi Moore's in* G.I. Jane, *but in the dream my hair was long and thick and curled. . . . I was not afraid of the scorpions although I was aware of their deadly stings.*

This dreamer is *really* having a bad hair day.

The story of Medusa is one of the classic Greek myths. She is an ugly customer: so ugly, in fact, that anyone who looks directly at her face is instantly turned to stone. Her hair is a mass of writhing, poisonous snakes. Hair is an ancient symbol of power; it is also a symbol of self. Do you know the biblical story of Samson and Delilah? Samson falls victim to his own failings and is undone by the treacherous Delilah: she cuts his hair, the apparent source of his immense strength.

Like Medusa, our dreamer's hair writhes with unpleasant things. In real life she has cut her hair short, but in the dream it is rich and full of vitality. The bad news, of course, is that it's also full of scorpions. When you put the two together you have to wonder about how this woman expresses herself. Perhaps the dream is telling her something she needs to know about how she acts in the world. She is not afraid of the scorpions, even though they are deadly and sting. In other words, she is in some way accustomed to them—they are part of her. Like Medusa, caution may be needed around her.

The person who suffers most from this bizarre hairdo is the dreamer herself. She is constantly stung. Even if she is a sweet person in outer life, the dream suggests she carries within herself the seeds of destructive and self-damning behavior. Perhaps she would benefit from finding ways to safely express her "scorpion" energies.

## IF YOU DREAM OF INSECTS AND/OR PESTS

- What kind of insect or pest is it? Sometimes that can tell you something about the real nature of the problem.
- Where are the insects or pests? The location tells you something. Some examples (remember these are broad generalizations):
  1. the kitchen may have to do with nourishment and nurturing oneself;
  2. the bedroom with comfort, rest, sickness and sexual issues;
  3. the living room with "where you live," i.e., the way in which you go about your life;
  4. the bathroom with needing to eliminate or let go of something, or express something;
  5. the garage with the vehicle of your life (work, home, etc.) or how you "store" things;
  6. the front yard with how you present yourself to others;
  7. the backyard with unconscious issues yet to be seen for what they are.
- What are the insects or pests doing? They could be attacking, running around, looking at you, in your hair—their actions are part of the message.
- What are you doing? Are you squashing them, running from them, spitting them out, watching them, playing with them, getting bitten by them, annihilating them—the action tells you something about how your inner resources are dealing with the issue.

Please use this list as a starting point for understanding—don't get locked into one idea only, but let your imagination flow freely. Any list like this can only start you thinking, because you have your own personal relationship with the images of your dream.

# 4

# SPIDERS AND SNAKES

I hate spider dreams. Snakes have never been a frightening nightmare image for me, but spiders will do it every time. I can trace my fear of spiders back to childhood. I was about five years old, running around the large playground at my kindergarten school. It was a country setting with shrubbery and a few trees scattered about the playground. I was running full tilt between two large bushes when I came to a sudden, heart-stopping halt, face-to-face with the biggest spider I had ever seen. An evil-looking, glossy black widow hung fat and menacing in a web thrown between the bushes. The sun shone off the glistening black belly with its telltale red hourglass. My face was inches away from this horrific apparition. I literally froze in my tracks. Slowly I became capable of moving and slowly I backed away, afraid the spider would somehow leap out of its web and attack me.

Since that day I have never liked spiders, and they have always been symbols of paralyzing terror in my dreams. Just as I was paralyzed in life, in my nightmares about spiders I am likely paralyzed in the dream. Fortunately for my peace of mind, I haven't had one of these dreams in many years—but I still remember them!

Our life provides many of the images of our worst nightmares. When it's time for a nightmare, the dreaming self selects scenes from the vast storehouse of our life experience that make us take notice. Even when we have no personal experience of some frightening encounter with a snake or a spider, we always have access to countless psychic images and endless amounts of information gleaned from books, movies, television, stories and cultural traditions.

There is something about a spider that frightens many people. They bite. Some are poisonous. Some are too big—they look like they can jump out and attack you. Some seem too ugly, too misshapen. In horror movies and fairy tales, spiders mean trouble, nastiness or danger. They are usually found in dark and unpleasant places, waiting patiently in their webs for prey. Have you seen *Raiders of the Lost Ark*? In the opening scenes Harrison Ford has to walk through horrible webs, huge tarantulas crawling on his back. We shiver as we watch.

Just as in real life, in our nightmares spiders spin webs—webs that can entrap us. Or perhaps we dream of spiders hanging overhead, waiting to drop on us. Spiders suck the juices from their prey, and in our worst dreams spiders represent something that feels like it is sucking the life right out of us. Spiders kill: they live by trapping and eating other kinds of life.

For men (and some women) spiders can represent something about women or a specific woman. That's especially true for the black widow, known for her poisonous bite and the unpleasant habit of devouring her mate.

*I recently broke up with my wife, just a few months ago. Now I dream of spiders almost every night—black widow spiders everywhere, crawling towards me, on the floor. . . . I pull back the bedcovers and my bed is crawling with spiders. I hate these dreams. What do they mean?*

In this man's dream it's a safe bet to say the spiders are making a statement about his failed marriage. He's angry and feels betrayed and attacked by his wife. One clue is the scene with the bed—the marriage bed, the bed of sexual union. Only now it's a bed full of spiders coming to get him.

To get rid of this dream, our dreamer has to look at his real feelings about his wife (and perhaps other women as well). He has to find a way to come to terms with them. Once he is able to let go of the anger and (probably) thoughts of inadequacy and helplessness he has about his ex, he won't need to have the dream anymore to prod him into doing something about it. The dream will go away. I think that this intense dream makes him a good candidate for professional counseling.

Spiders, like insects and scorpions, are a very old form of life. One of the things they represent in dreams is something primitive and basic—something rooted in the very depth of our being. There is not much in life more basic than the relationship with the mother. For someone who comes from a family where the mother was unloving, a spider can be a perfect dream symbol. The evil mother becomes an evil spider in the dream. Whenever the mother relationship is not good it sets up a wide range of problems for the unloved child. Those problems show up years later as nightmares, when we are older and better equipped to deal with the frustrations and pains of an unhappy childhood. Unfortunately, we don't usually know what a nightmare is trying to tell us. We just get frightened or upset and do our best to forget about it.

It's not only women who get turned into spiders in our dreams. Spiders can symbolize an evil male force as well. Someone hated and deemed evil, like Hitler, might be portrayed as a spider. If you saw a political cartoon of Hitler depicted as a spider, perhaps grasping helpless victims in his web, you would clearly understand it; it would require no explanation. In our dreams it can be the same. The spider represents some ensnaring and controlling force. It could be an overbearing boss; it could be a man who has a large and negative role in our life. It could be a father or a lover, but whoever it is he is sensed on the inner level as dangerous and menacing, with intent to do harm to us. Often the inner eye sees more clearly than the outer, and tries to warn us when we are in too deep.

If you are in a relationship unsettling to you and you have a spider dream, think carefully about what is taking place. Are you fooling yourself about the other person? Is he (or she) what he appears to be? Something in you may be warning you, or something may be stirred up by the power of your emotions. Honor your instincts and feelings. If they are shouting danger, maybe you should turn away. It's your call.

If you are having spider dreams, look on the bright side—at least you are not dreaming about snakes!

## *Snake Dreams*

Snakes get a very bad rap in our society. They have a fundamental cultural association with evil. You probably know the Garden of Eden allegory. It is Satan in the form of a snake who tempts Eve to eat the apple. It is the snake that is condemned by God to live on its belly in the dust. It is the snake that becomes the universal symbol of evil in Western tradition and religious teaching.

In the East people have a very good reason to fear snakes—they can kill you. You've probably seen an image of the mighty cobra, rearing up and spreading its hood, swaying in hypnotizing rhythm before its helpless prey. From the jungles of the Asian subcontinent to the rain forests of South America, from the southern coast of the United States to the southwestern desert, poisonous snakes are feared and hated. It's hard to find another image from nature (except, perhaps, spiders!) that can evoke such a universal reaction.

Along with spiders, *Raiders of the Lost Ark* also manages to get in a classic snake scene as well. Harrison Ford descends into a long-sealed Egyptian temple where the floor seethes with thousands of snakes. It's an image from his darkest dreams. "It had to be snakes," he says. It's funny to us in the audience, but not to him. He is acting out our shadow on the screen, forced to go through a truly nightmarish movie sequence before he breaks free into the light. The movie scene is an instant nightmare, but unlike our real nightmares it has no immediate meaning that must be unraveled and understood for our peace of mind. We can sit back and be entertained by scenes that would awaken us in a cold sweat if we were dreaming.

What do snakes mean in our nightmares? The answer is that it depends. It depends, for example, on our experience of snakes. If we were brought up to fear snakes, the stage is set for a nightmare image from our dreaming self. In this case, snake equals something that can harm us. Snakes are often thought of as slimy—part of their poor press, since this isn't really true. Snakes are cold-blooded, adding another layer to the sense of menace. We talk about people being "cold-blooded," or we say, "He's a snake," meaning he is not to be trusted and has bad intentions. When someone is more than a little crazy or dangerous, we say, "He has snakes in his head." So snakes are seen as evil, untrustworthy, dangerous and slimy. It's all the stuff of nightmares.

Snakes have other meanings as well. They have traditionally been a mystical symbol of wisdom and knowledge. It was this underlying, ancient meaning attached to the snake that carried over into the Old Testament, where eating from the Tree of Knowledge became an act of disobedience to God, with terrible consequences. Thus the snake, the symbol of knowledge, and Satan became one.

A snake in your nightmares, even though it may be terrifying, still carries that aspect of wisdom. It is a layer of the meaning. The snake is in your dream in order to teach you something you need to know about yourself, symbolically speaking. Are you with me? There is always an underlying aspect of the dream snake that has to do with self-knowledge and wisdom. It may not be earth-shattering knowledge, but it's something you need to know, nonetheless.

A classic interpretation of snake dreams is sexual. The dream snake is seen as phallic, a symbol of dangerous and forbidden sexuality. We're back to the Garden of Eden again, with its prohibitions against sexuality and knowledge of self. The phallic symbolism is an obvious choice—snakes penetrate into dark places, for example. We can have a snake dream sexual in nature and not at all nightmarish. We can have a snake dream where the sexuality makes us want to climb the walls in fear.

If you would like to see a kind of instant "dream" about snakes in the dark, sexual, dangerous and unconscious sense, there is a movie you can rent to illustrate what I'm talking about. The movie is called *The Lair of the White Worm*. It will never be nominated for any awards, but it is true to the symbolic imagery that appears in our nightmares. Be warned—this is most definitely not a movie for children or for the squeamish.

Even though many snake dreams are sexual in nature, it's important not to fall into the trap of thinking a snake is always about some sexual fear or desire. Here's an example of a dream that is ambiguous enough for the meaning to go in a couple of different directions.

*I've had a recurring dream involving snakes over the past few months. Last night I dreamt of a snake about to attack me and I viciously killed it by closing the back door on its head. I could see its fangs wide open towards me, so I slammed the screen door tightly and took off its fangs and part of its head. It was a scary dream, 'cause I don't like snakes to begin with, but I wonder what it could represent. I'm also not a violent person, so I was surprised at how I acted but satisfied about saving my life and protecting my family.*

The dream doesn't really give us enough information to say with certainty what the snake represents, but we can make some pretty good guesses based on what we already know. Sometimes dreaming of snakes alerts us to something going on in real life that hasn't yet surfaced into conscious awareness, like disease or a stressful and dangerous situation.

In this case, the dreamer feels attacked by something in her life. The fact this is a recurring dream tells us immediately that whatever the meaning, it's (1) important and (2) she isn't getting it. So it becomes necessary to have the dream again until the message is received. At least the mind hopes it will be received. There's no guarantee of understanding any dream.

She is surprised she acts so violently and slams the door on the snake. What do you think that means? She is "slamming the door" on what the snake represents. Her outer mind really doesn't want to know about it—it's too threatening. She is satisfied with the result, preserving stability and protecting her family. She makes the snake harmless, cutting off its fangs. Fangs can penetrate and poison.

By implication, the snake represents something threatening stability. Whatever it may be, her refusal to acknowledge it keeps the dream coming back to her. Perhaps she's considering an affair (the sexual aspect). Perhaps she's afraid of something in a sexual sense. By cutting off the fangs, she cuts off that penetrating aspect. That could be a sexual symbol.

Perhaps she's afraid of the knowledge of something her unconscious has already noticed but her outer mind refuses to look at. In this case, the fangs would represent the "penetration" of her consciousness by something she doesn't want to know about. The dream will continue until she resolves the issue or understands the meaning.

## UNDERSTANDING SNAKE DREAMS

If you have a similar dream, here are a few simple questions you can ask yourself to try and understand it. The first question seeks to reveal underlying sources of psychological and physical stress.

- Is there something going on in my life right now that makes me feel stressed and upset?
- What do I think of when I think of snakes?
- What does the symbol of a snake mean to me?
- Am I concerned about sex or a sexual area in my life? (Don't take yourself too seriously, but be honest—sex is a loaded subject, isn't it?)
- Is there something I am not letting myself see about my situation?
- Do I feel in charge of my life, or are things getting out of control?

This last question can be applied to the dream example given above. The dreamer slammed the door and cut off the snake's head. She asserted control. That might be exactly the wrong thing to do in real life, depending on the true meaning of the dream. "Family" could symbolize her entire inner "family" of self, adding depth to the importance of the dream. She must feel very threatened by something!

What do you do if you can't just slam the door on your dream snake? If the snake (or snakes) attack and begin biting you in your dream and you are unable to escape, then you can be sure things are getting out of hand. Here's an example:

*I hate snakes and have terrible nightmares about them. If I see them in a movie or on TV, I dream about them. Lately I've been having nightmares about being attacked by snakes. They bite me and leap up at me, and when I grab them they twist and sink their fangs into me. I can't get away from them.*

It's another dream of helplessness. Something is overwhelming the dreamer, and he is unable to overcome or meet it successfully. He can't get away from it. He wrestles with the snakes, just as he is wrestling with choices in outer life that feel threatening to him.

Snake dreams can sometimes foreshadow or warn of health problems. If you have a recurring dream like this example, you might think about getting a checkup. It's possible for snakes in a dream to represent serious disease, but if you dream of snakes it doesn't necessarily mean you are sick! That is only one possible interpretation.

You can see that spiders and snakes in nightmares alert us to psychic distress. Some part of us is really upset about something if we have a snake or spider dream. Nightmare images always represent something we fear. Often the meaning is hard to understand because the roots of fear may not be apparent. Tracking down the meaning of a nightmare is a little like standing in a hall of mirrors. Which reflection is really you? By setting your fear aside and taking a calm, reasoned look at the dream, you can find out.

# 5

## PARALYZED WITH FEAR—HYPNOGOGIC DREAMS

Have you ever had a strange and terrifying dream where you are paralyzed and can't wake up? Worse, have you thought you were actually wide awake, but unable to move a muscle? Meanwhile, strange and sinister shapes and people move about the room, voices and laughter are heard, perhaps it feels like someone is standing behind you or sitting down on the bed. Everything seems intensely real, but you are completely helpless. Such an experience is genuinely horrifying. People who have one of these often wonder if they are going crazy, especially if it happens more than once.

No, you are not crazy. You have entered what is called a hypnogogic (*hip-no-go-jic*) state. A neurological mechanism in our brain temporarily disables voluntary muscle movement during dreams. If such a mechanism did not exist we would physically act out our dreams, leading to injury or death. For some people this mechanism shuts down, leading to a serious result called REM sleep disorder, the technical name for what happens during sleep-walking.

While sleepwalking results from failure of the paralysis mechanism, hypnogogic states occur while the paralysis is fully turned on. When we experience a hypnogogic state, we are actually asleep. Because of the dream-triggered paralysis, we cannot move or cry out. It's a kind of awful waking dream, where somehow we have gotten out of step with the usual sleep patterns and become aware of our paralysis in a frightening and disturbing way. We are asleep in a nightmare where we can't move, believing we are awake.

As with many sleep and dream states, hypnogogic states are not well understood. They seem to occur when we are very tired or run down and are overstressed by our lives. Stress is always a factor in any kind of nightmarish state. People often report having one of these horrible nightmares when they lie down for a nap. It seems to coincide with entering a regular dreaming state (REM sleep), but something goes wrong.

Here are some examples of hypnogogic dreams. If they sound familiar, you probably need to take a look at how your life is going, in terms of stress, rest, satisfaction and relaxation. I feel strongly that hypnogogic states are a sign we must pay immediate attention to both our physical and mental well-being.

*I've had these dreams for many years; they are very intense. Usually there are many voices laughing or sometimes one voice. But this is very loud in my dreams. A lot of the time I realize where I am, but I am filled with panic and cannot move. It feels like I am being pulled from life. This continues until I am woken, usually by someone else.*

*I often dream, usually when I nap longer than an hour, that I can't open my eyes. I know I am dreaming; I can hear things going on around me. I just can't open my eyes or wake up. When I finally do wake up, I feel as if I had been drugged.*

The "drugged" feeling is very typical. We wake from such a dream feeling exhausted and leaden. Take a look at this next example and see if it's like your experience.

*I had a dream, which I can't remember, and I thought I had woken up. I felt all fuzzy, and I was thinking, "Am I awake?" I walked to the bathroom and I heard laughter all around me. I started yelling, "I'm not awake!" The laughter wouldn't stop. I knew I was dreaming but I couldn't wake up. It was so scary. I've been having dreams where I can't wake up lately. What does this mean and why was there laughter?*

Laughter, often ominous laughter, seems to be a part of many hypnogogic dreams. Over the years many people I've worked with have reported evil laughter when describing this kind of nightmare. Perhaps there is some part of our psyche that uses such chilling sounds to get our attention. It's one of the reasons people begin to think they are going crazy when they have these dreams. You can see why. Imagine that you think you are awake and find you can't move—and to top it off, there are strange voices and demonic laughter around you (in your bedroom, no less!) and you are helpless to deal with it. Some hypnogogic dreams are brought on by illness or medication.

*This dream occurred just after I had been ill in the hospital. I was on Demerol, but I dreamed I could hear my husband trying to call me and I couldn't see. Then I couldn't move. He shook me and I couldn't talk. His voice faded out as he shook me. I was stuck in a dark body and couldn't communicate. I prayed to God that I didn't want to die yet and I did wake up. I cried for a long time but can't get this out of my mind.*

A dream like this is awful—it seems so real and the dreamer feels so helpless. The feeling usually disappears when we wake, but if the dream is powerful enough we are left with emotional residue that cannot be denied. The woman who dreamed this dream experienced something akin to death, and felt like she really was dying. I would have trouble "getting this out of my mind" also. Such a dream brings us face to face with our fragile mortality and all the emotions that go with separation from loved ones. We fearfully connect to a sense of our own, inevitable extinction.

Like many important things in life, the way to deal with

dreams of paralysis or dreams where you can't force yourself to wake up is simple and complex at the same time. Simple, because you have both the ability and the inner resources to do what is needed so you don't have similar dreams in the future. Complex, because such dreams usually imply something needs to change on a fairly significant level.

For example, suppose an underlying cause of your hypnogogic dreams is the kind of job or work you are doing. Again and again I see people who are caught up in a cycle of work and stress that simply leaves them little or no time to rest and enjoy their life. If I point out to them that their comments show work is part of the problem, they almost always agree and then go right on to tell me why it can't be changed and nothing can be done about it. Yet the cure may lie in doing the very thing they say they cannot do! That's what I mean about simple and complex at the same time.

Don't sacrifice yourself on the altar of your work. Take time to relax, time to enjoy life. What good is it going to do if you succeed at the expense of your health and peace of mind? Dreams of evil laughter in your room while you lie helpless are a sure sign things have gone too far and that you need to bring some balance back into your life. Whatever the cause—work, relationships, financial stress, illness, family pressures or events, or any of the other ongoing causes of tension and stress in our lives, you can effect some change and give yourself some relief. Do it, and your dreams will refresh you rather than leaving you groggy and confused.

Sometimes it's not so easy to see the causes of stress or upset that are contributing to the nightmare. The person who related this next dream was not aware of anything particularly stressful going on in his life at the time. His dream occurred when he was drifting off—which is frequently when hypnogogic dreams appear.

*I've had this dream twice and it's really freaky. I'm not sure if I was totally asleep or just on the verge of falling asleep, but I know it only lasted a few minutes. In my dream it's like reality—I'm in bed but I'm awake and I feel paralyzed. I open my mouth to yell or scream, but no sound comes out.*

*I can't move either and I totally panic and try to wake myself up, but this is hard. When I come out of the dream, it feels so lifelike that it doesn't even feel like a dream.*

*When I had this dream the second time I was in bed again, but I felt like I was drowning, even though there was no water or anything that might obstruct breathing. I felt the panic, paralysis and likeness to real life again. I'm not sure whether I died or not.*

It's so easy to confuse dreams and waking reality. This dream adds a nightmare touch of suffocation and drowning. The feeling of suffocation comes because of the muscle paralysis accompanying dream states. He's still breathing, of course, but he can't consciously take a breath—that requires voluntary muscles, and they aren't available to him until he fully awakens.

## IF YOU SUFFER FROM HYPNOGOGIC DREAMS

- Take an honest look at your life situation. Chances are you are under severe stress for some reason. What can you do about it? Make needed changes.
- You can learn techniques for stress relief. Part of the stress pattern is the feeling that it is not possible to make changes. This is a normal feeling when caught up in a pattern of stressful behavior. In fact, change is always possible. If you are unable to cut workloads or effect some external circumstance, like a difficult relationship, try using meditation, biofeedback, exercise, improved sleep practices or anything else that lessens your mental load.
- Take time to refresh yourself and provide a counterpoint to your usual routines and habits. Perhaps you can't take a vacation, but you can find time to do something different and out of the ordinary. Go to a museum and look at paintings or take a walk in the country. See a movie or read a book. Rent old comedies with W.C. Fields or Laurel and Hardy. Listen to beautiful music for an hour. All of these things provide needed balance.

In the end it's up to you. Find a way to reach beyond the stress of your daily obligations to something relaxing and uplifting to your spirit and your dreams of paralysis will vanish.

# 6

# RUNNING FOR YOUR LIFE

Sooner or later, most of us dream about being chased—it's the most common theme in nightmares. These can be very frightening dreams. We know terrible things will happen if we are caught by whatever is coming after us. Murder, rape, torture and horror are only a few, closing steps behind. Why do so many people have these dreams? What do they signify?

Imagine you could go back in time, back to the primitive days of our caveman ancestors. Thousands of years ago life was short and dangerous: we shared the land with large, powerful and speedy beasts of prey. Saber-tooth tigers, giant bears and huge wild pigs could tear a human to pieces in an instant. The only defenses were to stand and fight or run. Life depended on luck and speed; all too often the chase ended in defeat and a horrible death.

Our brain still contains areas dominant during the earliest stages of human development. These parts of our brain respond instinctively to danger and stress, sounding the alarm and preparing us for flight or battle. Fear and danger trigger the instinctive response; the urge is to run, run faster than the thing that is after us.

Today there are usually no tigers outside our door but there are plenty of new threats and dangers to take their place. Our dreaming self still calls upon ancient memories of the chase and death. Instead of tigers and bears (although these can show up!) we dream of angry and relentless dark figures pursuing us with malicious intention.

There are many possible reasons for having a chase dream but fear, stress or insecurity of some sort will always be a factor. Often chase dreams are repetitive, occurring again and again over a long period of time. Sometimes the dreams are exactly the same, sometimes the scenes or characters change but the theme and results are the same. Here's an example of this kind of dream:

*In the last three years I have been having a repeating dream where I am running for my life. In one dream I was being chased by a group of people and I was jumping from building roof to building roof. In each dream I'm being chased by someone and I do things like Superwoman. Tonight I was in my house being shot at by a man at my front door. I knew the man in my dreams, but it wasn't someone I know in my real life. I am never hurt in my dreams, but they leave me very shaken when I awake.*

This dream is fairly mild—nonetheless, this woman wakes up "shaken." It qualifies as a nightmare. To make sense of the dream it helps to know something of her background and current life situation. What's going on, at home, on the job, at play? Perhaps by looking at her external, waking world the underlying stress causing the nightmare can be discovered.

In waking life our dreamer has a lot on her plate. She's a single mother of two in her early thirties. Her high-pressure job is very stressful, although she says she "enjoys it." She is still living at home, renting an apartment in her parents' house. She is applying for a new job and wants to start over in another part of the country. Does this sound a little bit like "Superwoman" to you? It does to me, and it's not that unusual a situation. Today more and more women (and men) are called on to perform feats of work and family that might be called heroic. Two kids and a tough job, plus the unresolved stress of a job search and a potential big move create a good psychological setup for a nightmare.

Male figures are the most common culprits in chase dreams. Without getting too far into the mysteries of dream symbolism, it's not hard to see male figures as representing all of the negative or positive qualities of men in general. In nightmares where we are chased by men or attacked by them, you can bet it is not a reflection of their positive side!

Some of the negative qualities of male dream figures include dominating authority, aggressive sexuality, physical brutality and shadowy portrayals of rigid or linear ways of thinking and doing things. Since the dream is an expression of our unconscious and personal self, the negative male figure represents some quality or combination of qualities or some fear within us.

In this case, I think the dreamer is looking at a reflection of her lifestyle and the choices she's made to support herself and her children. She works in a brokerage. It's demanding and linear work, fact-filled with a constantly changing informational context. Change happens very quickly and a mistake can cost a lot of money and trouble for her and for others. It's a masculine, high-pressure environment.

Unfortunately, there is a price to pay. She succeeds at the expense of time to relax and renew herself in ways nurturing to her feminine side.

## Male and Female Figures as Symbols

The symbols of masculine and feminine characters in nightmares (and in dreams of all kinds) are open to broad interpretation. It often depends on who, exactly, is doing the interpreting. It's not possible to say that male and female or masculine and feminine characters always mean something similar. Even so, we can make broad distinctions based on the way the characters act and on a concept of what feminine and masculine might mean as abstract concepts within our dreaming mind.

Here is a basic framework for understanding masculine and

feminine symbols I have used with good success in years of look-ing at dreams. In the abstract, masculine characters can symbolize something ordered, structured and mental. Feminine figures tend to represent something chaotic, natural and feeling-oriented. This is a very broad generalization, but it's a good place to start. Any of these broad qualities can have positive or negative connotations and either male or female figures can take on qualities of the other, depending on what happens in the nightmare.

When we look at the dream example above, using this frame-work gives us a clue about why these nightmares are visiting our dreamer. Her work is extremely masculine and detail-oriented, her life by necessity structured and organized. Think of her responsi-bilities as a single mother and all of the other stresses she deals with daily. The chase dreams reflect the inner stress and her "heroic" efforts to deal with it—she has to act like Superwoman in order to cope, leaping over buildings and staying ahead of her pursuers.

The man at the door shoots her: it's an image of masculine pen-etration. In the dream she "knows" him, even though he isn't anyone from real life. He is the mirror of her inner stress, some-thing she "knows" intimately, a part of her daily existence. The dream repeats, with variations, because she has not yet achieved the necessary balance in her life that could reduce all that stress. What is chasing her is her own way of doing things, and the dreams will likely continue until she makes some adjustments.

To understand what our dream-mind wants us to know, we have to make a leap in our thinking from the literal (there's a man who might hurt me) to the symbolic (there is something bother-ing the heck out of me and I need to figure out what it is).

Just to confuse things a little, it is sometimes true that a night-mare will use the symbolic to warn about the literal. If you are actually in a life situation where someone is posing a real threat to you, you could dream about that person. If you have such a dream, think about what you need to do. Are you in an abusive domestic situation? Is someone harassing you in some way? Take steps to protect yourself. You do not have to put up with it.

Often our dreaming mind will warn us of danger or upset

before a threat comes to our waking notice. We can feel threatened by so many things—illness, financial stress, a domineering boss (man or woman), an offensive co-worker, a demanding customer, an abusive relationship or even something we hear on the evening news. Unpleasant and threatening people show up in chase nightmares because they symbolize our feelings of helplessness and vulnerability—we can't control how they act and make them stop harassing us.

## Murderers, Rapists and Knives

Chase dreams often feature unknown assailants who pursue us for some unknown reason and threaten to harm us when they catch us. Here's one:

*For years now I have had so many dreams about people chasing me and trying to kill me. This one dream in particular scared me the most; it was very graphic and gory. I was being chased by a murderer who had already tried to rape me. He was carrying a large knife. All of a sudden I came upon a wall and couldn't run anymore. As soon as the murderer tried to attack me, another man tried to stop him. The murderer took his knife and slit the other man's throat—this is what was so gory. I remember exactly what his throat looked like, there were tons of blood and I could even see bones sticking out of his neck. Anyway, the murderer ended up catching me, but then I woke up. . . .*

The murderer/rapist is a classic figure in chase nightmares. He embodies all our fears of death, mutilation, violation and helplessness. Often he appears carrying a large knife. It is frightening to think about being stabbed and cut. Aversion to the sight of our own blood is rooted in our primal mind. That is one reason so many horror movies feature knives, axes or other awful instruments for cutting up helpless victims.

For years this woman has been chased by people trying to kill her in her dreams. That tells us whatever is bothering her is long-standing and deep-seated, perhaps going back to her childhood.

The dream is trying to get her to understand the problem in a general sense. Then she might be able to do something about it, based on seeing something about the nature of the difficulty. There is a big clue about the problem in the dream, although no solution is presented. Do you know what it is?

The clue is the wound to the throat. More than a wound, it is a horribly gory and specific image, really the key image of the dream. The murderer kills her would-be defender by slitting his throat. What is the throat, as a symbol? What do we do with the throat? We eat, we breathe—and we speak. It's a dream of severely wounded self-expression. This dreamer is unable to adequately express herself in the world in some fundamental way and it is tormenting her.

Her own "masculine" aspects, represented by the murdered rescuer, are not powerful enough or well enough developed to protect her from the violating, negative male force. It could be something to do with her father or another man; it could be a reference to all of the negative and critical influences in her life. Whatever the murderer represents, the result is the same: she is unable to fully reveal and express herself in her life. She is "up against a wall," seen in the dream when she reaches the place where she can run no further.

There is news of underlying strength in the dream—the murderer tried to rape her in the past but failed. She's managed to keep some core resistance alive within her, a refusal to let herself be completely overwhelmed by whatever the attacker represents. It's a good sign for potential change. To get rid of these dreams, she needs to do whatever it takes to reclaim who she is in a natural and fulfilling way. If she begins to do this, the dreams will eventually disappear.

## Bathroom and Toilet Dreams

I've seen a lot of chase dreams where the dreamer runs into a bathroom to hide. Most of the people I talk with think they are dreaming of a toilet because they actually need to go to the bathroom—they wake up and do need to get out of bed and relieve themselves. That is sometimes true, but if you combine a toilet with a chase, something else is going on.

What's going on is pretty simple on the surface: there's a need to let go of something, some idea or activity, concept or belief. A toilet is a pretty good symbol for letting go, don't you think? Moreover, it symbolizes letting go of something no longer needed—waste, in effect. If you are uncomfortable thinking about toilets and waste, you are like most people. It's a taboo subject in our society, which makes it a very effective dream image. Toilets can also appear in health dreams, but in chase nightmares they often refer to the need for getting rid of something, usually a belief or a perception.

*I am running from people who are after me. There are two or three men in dark business suits. I didn't do anything wrong, but they are trying to catch me for something—I don't know what. They are working together to try to corner me. I run into a subway train station. I can hear the commotion behind me as the men get closer.*

*Suddenly I see two women working at a newspaper stand. There is an open door behind their counter. I tell them I need to use their washroom desperately. I don't really need to use the washroom; I just use this as an excuse so I can hide from the men trying to capture me. I don't want to tell the ladies I am hiding from these men, because I don't want them to get frantic and accidentally give it away that I am in hiding. While hiding, I can hear and visualize the men wondering where I went. It was as if I had vanished and they couldn't figure out where I was.*

*While I was hiding I felt the urge to actually use the toilet and when I did I woke up. I know in the dream that I didn't do anything wrong, just like in the last dream I had of running away from people who were a threat to me.*

Notice that this dreamer repeats the theme that she "didn't do anything wrong." That's a clue—she must actually think, deep down, she has done something wrong! It doesn't have to be something specific. In fact, it is probably a very general feeling that she is wrong just because of who she is. It's a dream of self-worth and self-esteem.

The threatening characters coming after her are male, dominating, organized and business-like. That's why the dark suits appear. Business suits are a typical symbol of male authority and (often) anti-feminine thinking and perception. Many women are pursued in their nightmares by figures in suits.

She runs underground, into a subway station. The subway is something "underground," out of sight, unseen. She hides in the public toilet. That's the clue for needing to let go of something. She conceals her need to hide from the women at the newsstand. A newsstand is a place where we get news, information we haven't heard before. So these women, and the toilet behind the stand, symbolize something that is "news" to her. OK so far?

Why hide the truth from the women? The answer is that they represent an uncomfortable point of view for her. It's her dream; everyone in it is a symbolic representation of herself. If the dream is trying to say something about her relationship with male authority, then perhaps the women symbolize a part of her that is not comfortable acting on an equal basis with men. She might not want to admit that to herself in waking life.

In fact, she felt this was an accurate interpretation of the dream. What she must let go of is a false perception of herself as inadequate and wrong. What's required is no less than a redefining of herself as a woman, independent of the judgments and criticisms of unenlightened male thinking. Does this sound familiar?

## When Women Chase Men

This sounds like a great title for a comedy about sex. It is anything but funny to the man who has a horrifying nightmare of relentless pursuit. Just as the many issues women have with men show up in their worst nightmares, the same is true for men and their issues with women. Perhaps someday we will all live in a world where both men and women are nurtured and appreciated equally, but that time is not yet. Until then we will have dark dreams reflecting our deepest fears and insecurities about the opposite sex. This next example is a classic.

*I am in a dark and dangerous place: I know that something awful is going to happen and I can't seem to find my way out of the place I'm in. I'm naked and afraid. Suddenly a large man, also naked, bursts into the room. He has a long, evil-looking knife in his hand and he begins chasing me—I know he's going to kill me.*

*I run away, frantically running through a series of rooms. I can hear him crashing along behind me, gaining on me. I run into another room, but there is no way out. He starts towards me. He is very strong and powerful; I know I am helpless to stop him. Suddenly a woman dressed in red enters the room. She looks relentless. Her eyes seem lifeless. She also has a very large knife. She is overwhelming. She attacks the man and kills him—blood is everywhere, all over me, all over the room. Then she turns to me. I know that if I couldn't stop the man from killing me, I have even less of a chance against this woman. I know she has no mercy. She is inhuman, completely unstoppable and powerful. She comes toward me. I scream and wake up.*

This grim and significant nightmare is the kind of dream that would set a psychoanalyst to pulling out his notepad and muttering, "Hmmm," into his beard. There is severe distress in this man's inner world. How would you feel if you had this dream? I don't know about you, but I would be pretty upset.

It's bad enough to be chased relentlessly by a vicious male figure who can't be stopped and who will kill you if he catches you. It's worse to find that even this ferocious image hasn't a chance against a dead-eyed woman in red. This is a dream of serious inner conflict. In fact this man was going through a period of agonizing self-reflection and doubt. He was drinking heavily, had financial problems, and was feeling out of control and vulnerable in his life. In a way his own masculine forces had turned against him, threatening to overwhelm him. That is why the powerful, murderous man appears in his dream.

The woman in red is an even bigger problem. She is clearly more powerful, more relentless, more terrifying than the murderous man. She represents a very skewed relationship with the feminine (and by extension, with all women). For this dreamer the roots of the conflict were found in his negative childhood relationship with his mother.

I call dreams like this one "initiatory," meaning they signal the possibility of change and the start of an inner, psychic journey. Confronted in our dreams by something absolutely terrifying, unstoppable and destructive, we may be on the verge of new possibilities in our lives. It's as if we must die to something so we can learn to live in a new and more fulfilling way. If you have such a dream, count it as a blessing in disguise, perhaps preparing you for significant change and new potential in your life. Use the information in this book to help you unravel the meaning, and then move confidently to make whatever changes may be needed.

## WHEN YOU HAVE NIGHTMARES OF BEING CHASED

- Try to identify what is "chasing" you in real life. Something is overwhelming you in an emotional, mental or physical sense. It could be anything from work to relationship.
- Think about what you can do to alter things once you get an idea of the cause. For example, if you are caught in an abusive relationship, seek advice. There are always free counseling options in any town or city of moderate size, but they won't do you much good if you don't use them.
- Chase dreams signal ideas of helplessness and feeling at the effect of something. Do something to regain a sense of control over your life. It could be something as simple as re-arranging your day to include time for yourself to relax. It could be as complex as leaving a bad relationship or an unfulfilling job.
- Make sure you are doing everything you can to take care of yourself. Get enough sleep, eat well, get some form of exercise, take time to step out of the rat race.

# 7

# DREAMING ABOUT THE DEATH OF A LOVED ONE

When someone we love dies in our dreams it's one of the worst kinds of nightmares. We wake with tears streaming down our face or gasping with fear, heart pounding. Almost always our thought is that the dream might come true. Because it seems so real the experience is as powerful as if it had actually happened. We are left with a feeling of shock that reminds us too directly of our fear. Love makes us vulnerable, and in our vulnerability lies the potential for loss and grief—a dark balance to the joy and happiness brought to us by the presence of a loved one.

Dreams of a loved one dying tend to fall into four broad categories, mostly about family members. These are dreams about our children (or grandchildren), dreams about our spouse or mate, dreams about a relative dying or about a relative who has actually passed on, and dreams about very close friends.

It's tempting to say such dreams simply reflect the fear of loss we all hold hidden in our hearts about the ones we love. On one level that's true, but like all other nightmares there is a larger meaning to look for.

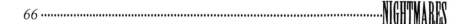

There is a mystery surrounding some dreams of loved ones who have already passed beyond. Though not always nightmarish in quality, they are disturbing to the people having them, who are left feeling grief-stricken and confused as a result of the dream. With these dreams, people frequently ask me if they are in contact with the person who has died. That is especially true for dreams where a loved one appears and reassures the dreamer all is well. Just in case you are a dreamer who picked up this book seeking help in understanding this kind of dream, we'll look at a couple of these later on in the chapter. They may not fall into the horrific category of nightmares, but they disturb and unsettle us just the same.

## *Dreams of Children Dying*

If you have a dream where one or more of your children dies, the first thing you must do when you wake is distance yourself from your emotional response. Begin by making an assumption that the dream, awful as it may be, is like any other nightmare. Something in you chose the images of the dream as the best way to communicate with your waking mind. From this point of view a dead child becomes another complex symbol used by the dreaming mind to convey a particular part of the message. One of the most difficult things about nightmares is their strong emotional content. It's hard to shift to the objectivity needed for understanding the dream.

There is a simple trick you can use to try and make sense of any symbol in any dream, including dreams of death and loss. The trick is to remember it *is* a symbol you are looking at. By definition, a symbol stands for something more than what it represents. It has an inherent quality that may or may not be immediately apparent. When your child appears in a dream, the meaning is complex. One useful concept is that the child is your offspring, an extension of yourself. In a dream your child usually represents something about yourself. Once you look at the dream from this point of view, the meaning may begin to emerge. Let's look at a couple of examples and I'll show you what I mean.

*I have 18-month-old twin girls. In this dream, I had filled up their crib with water for them to play in and put both of them in the crib. I then proceeded to go outside to water the yard and have a cigarette. As I was about to go inside, I saw my neighbor out in the front yard, searching for me with her son. I didn't want to talk to her, so I hid behind the wall and watched them search and give up after I didn't answer the door.*

*Then it occurred to me that I had to go upstairs to the babies—I could hear one of them playing but couldn't hear the other one. As I went up the stairs I thought something terrible had happened and started running to their room. When I went in my younger baby was facedown among all the clothes and toys in the crib—dead. I, immediately took her out of the water and started pounding on her stomach, scared out of my mind. Ironically, the first thing that occurred to me after the thought, "What have I done?" was "What will I tell people?" instead of "Is she okay?"*

*In the dream, every time I pressed her stomach in, water spurted out of her mouth, but to no avail. At least, not before I woke up in a completely terrorized state.*

*I have never left either of them in the bath alone, not to even mention the fact that I have yet to give them a bath together. My neighbor does bother me often, so my hiding from her wasn't so shocking . . . but I would never leave my girls like that!*

A chilling dream, isn't it? It is also a good example of how bizarre situations seem perfectly normal in a dream—like a crib full of water as a place to set children down to play. You can also see from her comments that the nightmare triggered a need to justify her care of her children, even though she is responsible and caring in waking life. That's a clue, suggesting she is secretly afraid she may not be a good mother. Anyone else reading this feel like that? I thought so—it's a normal feeling.

We know the dreamer doesn't really want to see her neighbor and finds her annoying in real life—she avoids her. The dream neighbor represents something she is hiding from, i.e., something she doesn't want to recognize on a conscious level. The dead baby represents something she's neglected. It's something vulnerable, placed at risk through inattention and unconscious behavior represented by the water in the crib.

The only way she can know exactly what the dream means is to ask what she has been neglecting or sacrificing in real life. It certainly carries a lot of emotional charge for her.

Here's another, brief dream with a similar theme.

*In my dream I was going somewhere and my daughter wanted to stay behind with the neighbor. When I started to look for her to let her know she could stay I could not find her. My cousin and I started looking for her all around the block; while searching we were joking and laughing.*

*Then we went inside my house and my cousin happened to look out the window and notice two children in the pool, under water. They appeared to have drowned and one was my daughter. Before it was confirmed she had drowned, I told myself to wake up because I didn't want to see my daughter dead.*

Another neighbor, another drowning. This time the child wants "to stay behind with the neighbor." In dream language it's like splitting off part of your self. What part? We don't know, and neither does she. She forces herself to wake up before she can confirm the death. That tells us she is not ready to understand what the symbol of the drowned daughter means: she doesn't want to know what it is. The child drowns in a pool; it's the pool of her thoughts and desires, emotions and fears. Laughing and joking in the dream while her daughter is drowning signals something inappropriate: something is not right in her waking life.

## Dreams of Projection

We see many things in our children. Our hopes and fears land squarely on them, along with our unexpressed vulnerabilities and our unresolved childhood experiences. In other words, we often don't see our children as they really are because we get caught up in our own issues. The name for this psychological reality is projection: it is an important concept for understanding nightmares.

Projection means just what it sounds like. We project our unconscious perceptions onto the broad screen of outer reality. That sometimes makes it hard to understand what is actually going on.

In nightmares the dream characters take on the projection, playing out for us a drama of emotions, thoughts and fears. In the theater of our dreams all of our unconscious fantasies, concerns, triumphs and defeats are displayed for consideration.

*I dreamed my five-year-old and three-year-old were dead. It was weird—I was crying in my sleep and I woke up with tears on my face.*

This dream reflects the secret fear of every loving parent. It's the kind of nightmare that occurs when we are under heavy stress, warning this dreamer of a need to nurture herself. It suggests she is unable to affect events in her life the way she wants. The image of losing her children means she is feeling unable to shape her life as she wants it to be.

If you have a dream about your children dying, think about the concept of projection. The dream children are reflections of your own, inner reality. Ask yourself if something is going wrong in your life. It might not be immediately apparent. These dreams always signal you are in some way neglecting an important part of yourself, perhaps simply forgetting to take care of yourself in a nurturing way. Too often we lose track of our inner needs and desires, sacrificing ourselves to routines of work, children, home and family. There's room for all of it, but it can take conscious desire and a determined effort to pull it off.

## *Dead Parents and Other Relatives*

What if you dream of parents dying or of a parent or relative who has already passed on? There are many cultures in the world where a dream about a relative who has died is thought to be an actual visit from the spirit of the deceased. It's not for me to say whether such things can happen or not. What happens after death is still a mystery, whatever beliefs we may hold about it. Personally,

I believe there is some kind of continuing existence after death and believe it is possible for the essence of loved ones to visit us in our dreams. However, I also think many dreams of someone who has died arise from our own unconscious as a way to help us resolve feelings and thoughts about the person who is gone. Whatever the truth may be, you can interpret such a dream from a psychological point of view with good results and genuine meaning.

## Dreams of Completion, Resolution and Peace

I often hear from people who believe a dead relative has visited them in their dreams, bringing relief and consolation or simply pointing something out to them. These dreams can bring completion, resolution and peace to the dreamer. They are important dreams, helping us come to terms with our loss.

*My father died in his sleep five years ago. It was a very sudden and unexpected death. Shortly after, I had a dream where he came to me in this very old and dilapidated house. We were very happy to see each other and he was smiling. I asked him if it were true that when you die you see a bright light. He just laughed (he always had a very hearty laugh). Then he guided me down through some rooms where the floorboards were falling apart, but we made it to the end. He then pointed to my husband, who was in a nearby room and sent me to him. I started to go toward my husband but looked back and my father was gone.*

A wonderful dream of resolution and integration! It signals a healthy shift in the dreamer's mind, addressing an important issue. The dream is about transferring trust from her father to her husband. The old house represents the outdated past, the structure underpinning her life before her father died. In other words, her father's passing left her in a transition period. She needed to make a shift from seeing her father as the primary male figure in her life to seeing her husband in the same way. Just because people get married doesn't mean they always make the change from seeing parents as being more significant than their spouse. Many a story has been written using this underlying theme.

When she asks her father in the dream about the bright light, she is symbolically accepting the fact of his death. Her dream-self is acknowledging that he has died, a necessary step for what follows. Acceptance is a key component in the grieving process: without, it the wound does not heal. In the house the floorboards are falling apart. The floorboards represent the "flooring" under her, i.e., the foundation of her life, in this case the support her father's presence provided for her. They are falling apart because he has died. She had not gotten past the shock of his death at the time of the dream.

Her father guides her down through the floorboards to her husband. It's an image of transition, signaling integration and acceptance. She has turned to the living, away from the past. When she looks back her father is gone, marking completion of the inner transition.

Did her father really come to her in a dream? Certainly he did in a symbolic way, and that is good enough. This dreamer still occasionally dreams about her father, and she says that she always feels good after waking.

Transition dreams about dead loved ones often present a healing message.

*My grandmother was widowed at the young age of thirty-eight. She remained single for four years, when she found a nice man whose wife had passed away. Immediately, the two were in love and got married. When they got married, my grandmother would have dreams in which her first husband talked to her. She says it was so life-like she could touch his hand. She had a dream like this about once a month. Finally she asked him (in a dream), "What are you doing here?" He replied, "I want to make sure you are happy, healthy and safe." "I am happy, healthy and safe," she replied. She then asked him if he would no longer visit her in dreams, because she was feeling guilty. She loved her new husband just as much as her last husband, and she felt awful having dreams about her first husband. The dream never happened again.*

That's a completion dream if I ever saw one, about coming to terms with the conflict inherent in loving two different men. It reflects the end of a time of inner adjustment, shifting loyalties from the first husband to the second.

I hope you can see you need not fear dreams about loved ones dying. They don't usually foreshadow actual death, although it's true there are times when actual death may occur. Those kinds of dreams usually involve someone known to be ill. Our unconscious mind picks up on subtle clues about the sick person and logically anticipates the end of life. Mostly, though, such dreams reflect concern for the people we love.

If you dream of a loved one returning to you, take a step back from any upsetting emotions. Chances are your unconscious is trying to help you come to terms with your loss. Embrace the dream in the spirit in which it is offered.

# 8

---

# $R$ APE AND ATTACK

Terror, helplessness and overwhelming fear of harm are common components of many nightmares. Rape meets all of those criteria. As a dream symbol, it signals the dreamer is feeling violated on a basic level of his or her being. Yes, men are raped in dreams also.

There is something so defiling about rape, so overwhelming and shattering to one's sense of self, that it makes perfect nightmare material. Rape dreams ought to force us to look at our lives very carefully, because something is going on that is as violating and destructive to our self-esteem as actual rape would be in real life. Whether dreamed by a man or a woman, dream-rape signals serious upset within. To be raped is to have all of one's personal boundaries trampled. Perhaps only murder represents a more fundamental indignity.

Sometimes people have dreams of being forced into sex with someone, but there is no upset in the dreamer's mind. Those kinds of rape dreams have a different meaning than the violent ones. What they have in common with the violent dreams is the underlying idea of union with something, for better or for worse. Sexual dreams are often a metaphor for joining psychically with whatever is represented by the dream partner. In violent rape dreams, the rapist represents something (or someone) that feels dangerous to one's mental and emotional well-being. It is sometimes hard to say exactly what that is—it's necessary to look at the details of the dream and ask some hard questions, seek truthful answers and then act on the information discovered.

There are so many ways we can become insecure in our lives that it is impossible to give one perfect interpretation for dreams of rape. The only thing we can say for sure about them is that some deep-seated anxiety or insecurity exists. We will be better off if we can identify it and assess it on a conscious level. After all, that is why our dreaming mind gave us the dream in the first place.

Here's an example of a rape dream trying to resolve feelings of shame and guilt, the result of an actual rape by a married man.

*About two or three months ago I was "raped" by a married man. The reason I say "raped" is that I didn't exactly say no to him, but it wasn't something I had a say on. It's a long story. . . . All in all I was afraid of this man and wasn't sure how to say no to him. After all this time I had a dream about him.*

*He and I were sitting on a couch with his wife across from us in a chair. We were all sitting around chatting as though we were the best of friends. He started to come on to me and all I could do was push him away. I kept asking him, "What are you thinking? Your wife is right there." He continued to try to kiss me and I continued to say no.*

*The next thing I know I am on the floor with him on top of me insisting that it is OK to kiss him . . . that his wife doesn't mind. I try to get him off me as he pushes himself into me . . . kissing me. All of a sudden, blood is coming out of his mouth. I quickly get up and ask him what is going on. Blood then starts to come out of my mouth.*

*The setting changes and I am bent over a trash can filled to the brim with vomit . . . my vomit. I am throwing up every couple of seconds into this trash can. In my sleep I can feel the vomit in my mouth and I can also smell it. I kept trying to cover my mouth and press against my lips to keep from vomiting. When I woke up my fingers were pressed against my lips.*

*I have never dreamt of this man before and have spoken to him only once since the incident. I don't understand why I would have this dream. I have never had one like it and thought I had gotten over it [the rape]. . . .*

Do you get a feeling about why she would have this dream? It's often a lot easier for someone else to understand something about a powerful dream than it is for the person who dreamed it.

The dreamer thought she had "gotten over" the rape, but the dream makes it clear she has not. She feels guilty: the man is married and she didn't "exactly say no." It is also clear she felt afraid to say no. I think many women reading these words know how she felt. Notice that a key component here is feeling powerless and unable to control a real-life situation.

Throwing up in a trash can seems like a pretty good image for feeling sick about the whole thing, don't you think? The blood in his mouth and in hers is a symbol of the violation she felt, showing how her psyche has tied rapist and victim together. It is part of what makes her vomit. Blood symbolizes the psychic injury.

The dream is telling her she needs to do something to make herself feel better about the rape. I don't know what that is—she'll have to think it through. It could mean confronting the rapist, but if she couldn't avoid him in the first place, that doesn't seem likely at this stage. The best advice is probably for her to seek counseling and professional advice on how to handle her feelings of helplessness, anger and self-blame.

What about dreams of rape when an attack hasn't actually occurred?

*I have these recurring dreams of being raped. I've never been raped, or even sexually offended. I've had many dreams, but two stand out. In the first, I was in a home unfamiliar to me. My mother and father were in the dream. They slept in a room with two doors facing the living room. In between the two doors was a couch where I slept. The walls were of plywood and the couch was of old material, rough, brown. There were multicolored afghans on it. The room reminded me of one of my grandmothers' homes. Anyway, Dirk Benedict [the suave guy from* The A-Team] *came in and raped me. I don't remember my feelings during the dreams, except for betrayal, fear and confusion.*

*A second dream was far scarier! It was so real! It happened in my own bedroom. In the dream I woke suddenly and the two doors in my room were both open (I keep them closed when I sleep). I could see everything in my room . . . I realized I was naked and had just been raped. I was so tired, though, I could not keep my eyes open. I fell asleep. An overwhelming fear grew inside me, even as I slept in the dream. I woke suddenly again, but I had a very hard time opening my eyes (in the dream). This time it was before the attack. I could hear the person walking in the adjoining bathroom. I could hear the handle rattling. The fear grew and I thought it would make me explode, but I was helpless and again I grew so tired I fell asleep. This process of waking and hearing the attacker in the bathroom and then falling asleep occurred five or six times.*

*Finally, the last time, I struggled to stay awake. I could see the light under the door in the bathroom; I could hear the door handle rattling. I tried to yell for my mother but the sound wouldn't come out. I tried over and over, screaming at the top of my lungs. I woke for real this time, whispering, "Mom."*

*It was so vivid and real. I had not realized it was a dream until I woke for real.*

These dreams occurred to a young woman just coming into deeper awareness of herself. They reveal underlying insecurity about separating from her parents and her dawning concerns about sexuality. The common symbol tying these two dreams together is the two doors: the two doors of her bedroom and the two doors where her parents are sleeping.

Dirk Benedict is an idealized male figure. In the television show he leads a team of big-hearted and heroic misfits against villains of all kinds. He's a comic book type of character, clean-cut and tough talking, with high moral values. He protects the weak and innocent and is a champion for law and order. But he turns into a rapist in her dream! He has become a symbol for her expanding understanding of the real world. In the real world, there don't seem to be any Dirks around. In the real world, sex and sexuality are difficult issues that must be dealt with, and most men aren't going to be like Dirk. As a dream rapist he marks the end of innocence, at least regarding the subject of sexuality. The ideal male of her fantasies is symbolically transformed into a betrayer. The dream reflects growing recognition that real life and real sex may not be like the romantic stories she sees on television.

## REASONS WHY WE DREAM OF RAPE

Are you beginning to see how we can look at a few key images in a nightmare and then arrive at an idea of what the dream is about? If you have a rape dream, here are some reasons why you may have dreamed it, along with advice for handling the dream.

**Rape, crime or trauma.** Victimization of any kind, including actual rape, physical trauma or violent crime, can set the stage for rape dreams. The best advice I can give you is to seek out help and support for getting through the feelings. There are usually victim advocate programs and free counseling available in most large towns and cities. Contact your local police department or look up county and city services for counseling.

**Relationship problems.** If your relationship has gone bad, especially if it is abusive and disrespectful toward you, rape dreams may start to appear. What to do about it depends on your situation. It is never acceptable for one partner to physically abuse and attack the other. If physical abuse is an issue, seek professional advice and start thinking about how to leave the relationship. I cannot emphasize this strongly enough! If the problem isn't physical abuse but more along the lines of how you get on together, counseling may help. Whatever the problem, seek advice and take action, otherwise nothing is likely to change.

**Feeling helpless about something in your life.** A bad job situation, serious health problems with unsatisfactory or invasive treatments—anything that makes you feel completely helpless and not in control—may prime your dreaming mind for a rape nightmare. The solution is to regain the feeling that you can affect events and circumstances in your life. Perhaps you need to ask for better conditions or circumstances. If you make the effort to communicate your needs, it can produce results. Stand up for yourself and back yourself up, whatever the situation. Trust your feelings and validate them.

**Self-criticism and anger turned inward.** You can symbolically violate yourself by criticizing yourself unnecessarily and by suppressing anger. Intense anger needs some form of safe expression, and if it can't go outward it will turn inward. Counseling can teach you how to handle feelings of anger in a constructive way.

**Feelings of sexual inadequacy, ambivalence or frustration.** Sexual issues are so pervasive in life that problems can easily appear in our dreams. Dream rape can be a symbol of sexual dysfunction or uncertainty. There isn't any pat answer for problems centered on issues of sexuality. Sexual problems may be rooted in depression, physical complications resulting from illness, or any number of psychological possibilities. The best thing to do is talk with your doctor or another health-care professional.

**Unconscious desires**. By this I mean the unconscious wish to be violated, ravished, conquered or forced into forbidden territory. This is one of the darker areas of our human psyche, part of the shadow content we all carry within. Our unconscious desires often show up in our dreams and may take on nightmare form. It's not possible to address this area adequately here. You should know that such fantasies are fairly common and in themselves don't signal anything abnormal or wrong. It's only a problem if you think it is. If you harbor secret fantasies of violation, and if those fantasies disturb you, you might want to talk with a counselor or therapist about it.

## Attack Dreams

Attack dreams are similar to rape dreams because they reflect loss of control. They are different from rape dreams because the kind of violation is different, focusing more on fear of bodily harm and death. Both rape and attack dreams refer to an assault on personal boundaries and something very troubling to the dreamer. Attack dreams occur about as frequently for men as for women.

Often attack dreams occur when we are facing difficult change in our lives. The outer uncertainty creates an inner context of fear, and a dream appears to let us know the stress is becoming unacceptable. Here's an example from a woman dreamer, but a man could have dreamed it just as easily.

*Last night I had a dream that I was driving through a very crowded small town. There were people crowding the streets and heavy road construction that made it difficult to get around.*

*I noticed a man in a car behind me. It was the only other car on the road. I knew he was following me and wanted to hurt me. Because of increasing amounts of construction, it was harder and harder for me to maneuver—I had to stop for pedestrians more and more frequently. At one point I looked in my rearview mirror and the man that was following started screaming at me and yelling that he was going to kill me by ripping my arms off and then torturing me further. He kept yelling over and over about ripping my arms off. . . . I realized he was going to get out of his car to get me.*

*The road was barricaded—I couldn't go any farther in my car. I knew I was going to die very soon. A couple walked by my car and I begged them to get help. I told them the man behind me wanted to kill me. They both said that he would kill me—they knew it—and there was nothing anyone could do about it. At this point I woke up.*

If you had this dream, how would you get a handle on it? The answer is always the same. Pick out the key scenes and then try to get a sense of what they mean by letting your mind come up with associations for the images. In this nightmare several important images provide clues to the meaning—the follower, threatening to rip off her arms; the construction delays that make her vulnerable; the couple that tells her nothing can be done.

Construction is a good dream image for things torn down and built up within the inner self. We sometimes have to tear something down to make room for the new. That is the context of this dream. Something being built: a road, a path, and a way through life. Do you see how road construction can symbolize these things? The car represents her vehicle—herself, her body, and her way of doing things.

The crowds are an image of inner clutter and resistance to the changes. The killer will tear off her arms—that's about feeling powerless and ineffective. The couple represents a part of her inner self that knows the confrontation can't be avoided. She will have to go through whatever changes are coming, even if she does not want to.

The importance of the dream lies in understanding the implications. If she knows she is panicking inwardly and feeling helpless, perhaps she can do something to take charge of her situation. She doesn't have to be powerless, even though change seems inevitable.

Women often have attack dreams that feature a fiancé, husband or boyfriend attempting to protect them. Sometimes the male is able to ward off the attackers. That kind of dream could mean the dreamer sees the chosen man as a real protection in the outer world; it can also mean she is able to call on resources within herself to protect her. A dream where the lover or fiancé successfully fights off attackers could symbolize inner transition toward marriage and be part of the shift to seeing someone else as being intimately on your side.

Men sometimes dream of desperately fighting male attackers, often against overpowering odds. Just as with women, the trigger for such dreams is usually an unacceptable level of stress. The stress may be found in the competitive workplace, in an unsatisfactory relationship, or in any number of possible life situations where feelings of inadequacy and potential failure are lying in wait. Many men are not very skilled in expressing their feelings and concerns, especially if they think those concerns somehow reflect badly on their sense of self as masculine. If the thoughts and feelings are not expressed consciously, they will find a way to be expressed unconsciously. That can range from inappropriate aggressive behavior to screaming nightmares dramatizing the feelings of inadequacy.

## IF YOU DREAM OF BEING ATTACKED

- Don't panic! The dream may be terrifying but it's simply trying to get your attention about something.
- Ask yourself if there is any situation in your life that feels especially threatening in an emotional, mental or physical way.
- Talk about the nightmare with someone you trust—they may see something that you cannot.
- Think of ways to regain a sense of being in charge of things. Attack dreams always signal a feeling of being out of control.
- Take steps to assert yourself in constructive ways and make any changes that might be necessary.

It's important to remember that nightmare attack is a symbol of inner stress. Stress has a source that can usually be identified. Once you know what it is, you can do something about it. Make the effort. The payoff is better sleep and better health, not to mention the end of your nightmares.

# 9

# $B$UCKETS OF BLOOD

Nothing compares to the sight of blood. It's one thing if we are talking about a scratch or cut, but it's another story entirely when large quantities of blood are involved. Spilled blood is a vivid red reminder of our mortality and vulnerability, triggering thoughts of pain and death. It's bad enough looking at someone else's blood. How much more horrible, then, if the blood is ours?

Since the loss of blood can lead to death, blood in dreams stands for death as well as life. The two are are inseparable, and blood is a symbol for both. In the Western and Christian religious sense, blood represents redemption of life and spirit, through the torturous journey of Christ's passion and shedding of blood to redeem mankind. In Christian communion the wine consumed is symbolically transformed into the blood of Christ, signaling internalization of the spiritual teaching and faith in the Christian mystery.

All of the major religions and many lesser-known teachings recognize the importance of blood. Blood represents life, and life is tied in to the divine mystery, celebrated according to the particular forms and practices of the religion. Through blood sacrifice, sin and evil are redeemed. This collective, cultural meaning can show up in dreams. Bloody nightmares can signal a new beginning, an inner sacrifice with a potential for redemption and renewal.

In movies, blood is always a disturbing element. The appearance of blood in a movie always leads to unpleasant results. Psychopathic and supernatural murderers leap out to stab and hack their helpless victims to pieces; blood flies everywhere, and we cringe in our seats, unable to avoid the feeling of horror.

Whatever the impact of big-screen nightmares, it's nothing compared to a private and real nightmare that wakes us screaming. I think that of all nightmares, the ones filled with blood are the worst. Remember, to our minds the dream seems real. We may wake shuddering and grateful it was only a dream, but the experience is very disturbing. It should be—we are confronted with images engraved at the basic levels of our existence, a cellular awareness that screams at the vision of its own dissolution and destruction.

Blood dreams are serious dreams. They tell us something is very much amiss with our emotional health and well-being. They demand action and signal an underlying disturbance that must be recognized and dealt with to preserve or regain peace of mind. Here's an example:

*I've had this dream repeatedly since I was sixteen (I am now twenty-four). In this dream I find myself in a deserted house along with three other people—I have no idea who they are. We are searching for a way to get out. We find ourselves in a basement and we huddle together trying to figure a way to get out.*

*When we come to a decision to stay together, an evil voice begins to laugh. We look around for the source and see no one; then the lights go out. We hear running water. Then the lights come back on and we are standing knee-deep in blood. Needless to say, we all freak out.*

*The lights go back out and the evil voice shouts, "Only one will survive!" The people with me all begin to scream in pain. The lights come back on and I am alone. The blood is up to my chin. A severed arm passes in front of my face and I scream. I never get past this part. . . .*

Whoa! I don't ever want to have a nightmare like this, and neither do you! And this is a repeating dream, one going on for eight years and counting. No Hollywood scriptwriter could come up with anything much more horrible than this dream.

The problem represented by this dream is long-standing. In other words, it's a core issue and needs to be resolved. We know that because it has repeated for so many years. Something is really up for this dreamer; she needs to deal with it consciously or the dream will keep coming back.

The dream speaks of abandonment. The deserted house represents a feeling of desolation and isolation. It could be referring to an external situation and a feeling of abandonment from without; it could be referring to inner abandonment, meaning the dreamer has abandoned herself on some fundamental level. What does it mean to abandon yourself? It means to not back yourself up, to back down from what you feel is right, to submit when you ought to resist—you get the idea.

The other people in the dream are inner aspects of the dreamer that cannot survive the onslaught. The evil voice represents the essence of the problem. It seems determined to destroy yet promises "one will survive." That is the only shred of good news in this dream, because it implies that in spite of everything, she will come through the ordeal. After all, it's her dream and she is the "one" who is dreaming it.

The lights going on and off emphasize the unconscious nature of the problem. She's in the dark about things, not able to see the cause of the blood and screaming. Lights off—something terrible happens. Lights on—she gets to see the increasingly awful result. Finally she is up to her chin in blood, almost drowning. She sees an arm pass in front of her—a symbol of her helplessness and powerlessness. I'd scream too, wouldn't you?

In this case, I'd recommend counseling. It's not always needed, but a horrible dream repeating over years does signal an ongoing problem. Sometimes outside guidance opens the right door and relief can be found.

If you have blood dreams and see a specific wound, you can

sometimes get a very good idea of the general meaning of the nightmare by thinking about the nature of the wound. Each area of the body can have symbolic meaning revealing something about the message of the dream. Some of these meanings have even found their way into slang and general speech. For example, if someone gets "cut off at the knees," what has happened? You know what the phrase means—they've been completely disempowered. All nightmare dream wounds can represent inability of some sort in the real world; all symbolize some area of vulnerability in an emotional, physical, mental or spiritual sense.

To help you figure things out I've created a "symbolic wound" list with some possible interpretations. Please remember that these are very general interpretations. Since each person's dream is unique, the challenge is finding the actual meaning that applies to your situation. Use this list as something to stimulate your thinking.

## SYMBOLIC WOUNDS

**Feet:** Foundation, ability to move forward in the world, connection to earth (grounding, feeling grounded), connection to the intuitive aspects (earth/feminine), connection to sense of self (rooted in earth).

**Legs/Knees:** Support, movement, ability to escape, something crippling to you, feeling "stuck" in life, connection to earth (see above).

**Pelvis/Groin:** Sexual issues, issues of creativity and outward expression, sense of self as man/woman, power and self-empowerment, life force, relationship, desire to unify with something (idea, person, concept, etc.), union with something.

**Buttocks/Anus:** Sexual issues, power issues, elimination of something, vulnerability, issues of guilt and self-worth, where you "sit," the "seat" of things.

**Back:** Support, something unseen, something unconscious, vulnerability, fear of attack, inability to see what's "behind" you.

**Stomach/Intestines:** Nourishment, ability to "digest" or take in ("stomach") something, vulnerability and/or fear (the stomach and intestines are the most unprotected part of the body), something inside of oneself, the center of emotions, emotional as contrasted with mental.

**Chest:** Painful emotional wounding (the heart). Fear of death, feeling suffocated by something (lungs), feeling overwhelmed by something, feeling dangerously confronted by something, something in front of you (meaning you may not be seeing something right in front of you causing the nightmare), fear of something coming up for you (situation, change, etc.).

**Throat:** Self-expression, ability to communicate, creative expression, something "choking" you that "can't be swallowed," feeling threatened when you express yourself.

**Neck:** Could also be self-expression (see throat) but can represent the connection between the head and the body, *i.e.*, a wound can represent separation between heart and mind, feelings and thoughts.

**Head:** Mental approaches, thoughts and ideas, perception of things (see eyes), sense of self-identity and the way in which we think about life, mental as contrasted with emotional.

**Face (mouth, nose, eyes, forehead):** Self-identity, the way we present ourselves to others, expression (mouth), life energy (mouth, nose), something "smells" (nose), the way we look at things (eyes), not seeing something (eyes), intuitive or spiritual wounding or issues (forehead).

**Arms and Hands:** Ability to do things in the world, ability to effect change, ability to reach out to others, control (lack of it), helplessness, crippled expression in the world, frustration with something.

You can see there is a lot of room for different interpretations of any dream wound, including possible meanings not on this list. Even so, by looking at the image you can get a start toward making sense of what your nightmare is trying to tell you. For example, suppose you dream about someone (or yourself) having his or her head cut off. That would qualify as a nightmare, wouldn't it? Whatever else was going on in the dream, it would be a safe bet to look in waking life for a conflict between emotions and thoughts. In other words, the dreamer could be overriding important feelings about something because it seemed best from a logical point of view. Such a dream would mark this approach as a big mistake.

If you are drowning in blood, as in the dream given earlier, things have definitely gotten out of hand. So much blood is a sign that the problem (whatever it may be) is affecting your ability to function well in life. It takes a lot of mental and psychic energy to repress big issues in your psyche. A blood-soaked nightmare is a kind of psychic safety valve as well as a warning something needs to be done. If you have one blood dream, try to identify the source of distress in your life. The specific images of the dream may give you the clue you need to figure it out. If you are having repeating dreams awash in blood, please consider talking with a professional therapist. Those dreams mean something must be done for your peace of mind.

# 10

# FACELESS HORROR

*In my dream I am in my bed and just waking from sleep. My room is becoming light, as if it is early or pre-dawn. I have a sense of dread, as if some undefined, negative energy is surrounding me. I don't know if my husband is next to me or whether I am alone in the bed. As usual, it feels hard to breathe. I notice that the covers are pulled up off the bottom of my feet, leaving them exposed. Within seconds, a hand (the size of a human one) or paw that is black and hairy emerges over the end of the bed. I can see the pads under the twisted fingers as they firmly latch onto my toes and begin to pull me over the end of the bottom of the bed. I wake with a yell.*

This nightmare is straight out of our worst childhood fears. Do you remember? Is there something hiding under the bed, waiting to grab our little fingers and toes and haul us under to some terrible, dark place? It's all the more horrible because our bed is supposed to be a safe place, the place where we can let down our guard and sleep without fear. That's not the case for this dreamer.

A dream so powerful requires attention. This woman's sense of safety and inner security is threatened and she needs to take a hard look at her life to discover the cause. Her statement, "As usual, it feels hard to breathe," suggests the possibility of chronic illness as a cause—the monster at the foot of the bed could be a symbol of the illness and her struggle with it.

Sometimes we can't easily point to a specific cause for fear, like an abusive spouse or serious illness. It can be a subtle combination of things, built up over time and destroying our sense of well-being and self-esteem. Then counseling may be needed to unravel the knots and guide us back to a place in the light.

Nightmares of monstrous and faceless creatures and evil forces are nothing new. As long as there have been humans there have been dreams of demons, danger and darkness. Legends, myths and stories from all cultures and all times reflect our common human fears, taking shape in folktales as demons, goblins, trolls, witches and horrible spirits. All are dedicated to making life as miserable, frightening and terrible as possible for us poor mortals.

An unfamiliar and potentially dangerous situation can trigger a dream of faceless horror. This next nightmare came to a woman sleeping alone in a small cabin in Alaska, next to the forest. Deep, wild forest is one of the all-time favorite settings for terrible deeds in dark fairy tales. We may be a long time removed from the campfires of our ancient ancestors, but something in us has never forgotten the terrors of the dark and dangerous forest primeval. Modern movies and television shows still use the forest in the same way to create an atmosphere of horror. A good example is the popular *X-Files* television show, a weekly presentation of nightmares, many set in the mold-covered forest depths of the Pacific Northwest.

*I was asleep and was "awakened" by the sound of the door on the first floor opening and closing. I knew my husband was away and shouldn't be coming home at this time. I was listening carefully, and I was struck with deep fear because someone was in my house. The footsteps came up the stairs. . . . I couldn't move, even though I desperately wanted to get up and hide. . . .*

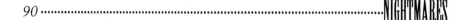

*I was watching the opening to my bedroom (the second floor was directly accessed by the stairs; there was no door) and I saw a large male (I assumed) figure come up and stand at the foot of my bed. It was a shadow, no features, just pure black. I wanted to scream but could not make my body do or say anything. Instead I made a very small squeak. I was sure that I was about to be raped and/or killed.*

*I could feel my heart trying to pound itself out of my chest. I tried to reason with myself while I was just looking at this shadow—it was doing nothing but standing at the foot of my bed. The next thing I knew, it was morning. I checked myself, unconvinced this had not been real, because it had been so real, and my awakening in the morning seemed so abrupt in relation to what I had seemingly experienced (from the dark of night and terror to the light of day and nothing wrong). Nothing was wrong with me and nothing had been disturbed in the house. The front door was locked.*

We don't have to look far to understand what sparked this dream. She was alone in the forest, far from help and neighbors, next to the unknown—in fact, right where dangerous and wild animals like the grizzly bear live, hunt and kill. Our dreamer was sleeping in a place where she felt vulnerable and unprotected. The shadow at the foot of the bed stands for all of her worst fears of rape, murder and violent death, brought on by the unfamiliar and unknown environment. Her helplessness in the dream reflects the underlying terror we feel when we are vulnerable and not able to ensure our safety.

Here's one from an eighteen-year-old girl who had some bad times around the time of the dream. She was beaten by her mother and left home with numerous injuries and a concussion. A month later she totaled her grandparents' new car in an accident and got another concussion to boot. A week after that the nightmares started, waking her screaming and dripping with sweat.

*I'm driving along during the day and listening to the radio when I get this feeling there is something really bad in the backseat and it wants to hurt me, even kill me. I slam the car to a stop and throw myself out the door and run. Somehow I fall to the ground, and then I feel claws starting to dig into me. I can't tell what it is, but it reminds me of a large cat, and it's ripping me to pieces. Then I wake up, and it still feels like I have marks on my body. I have to turn on the light just to check and convince myself that I am OK. In seven days I've had this dream three times. . . .*

How would you like it if something evil attacked you from the backseat of your car in real life? Like the dreamer in Alaska, this girl needs to actually check herself for injuries to make sure the dream wasn't real. That's how convincing nightmares can be. The events in this young woman's life set her up for the dream, bringing out all her insecurities. Add in two concussions and a lot of guilt about wrecking the car and we're well on the way to Nightmare City.

Notice the setting of the dream—driving down the road. Aside from the obvious connection we can draw because of her accident, driving is a symbol of control. But she is not in control any longer, at least as far as her dreaming self is concerned. The backseat is dream-speak for something unseen "behind" her, *i.e.*, something not yet conscious. In this case I think it's pretty much what it appears to be—vulnerability and concern about striking out on her own in a harsh and indifferent world. The solution lies in confronting her fears and regaining a sense of trust in herself. That might not be easy, but it can be accomplished with support and intention.

## Dealing with Dreams of Faceless Horror

If you have a dream of faceless horror attacking or approaching, what can you do?

- Remind yourself that nightmares are trying to tell you something, not just scare the wits out of you.
- Assume that there is something in your life bringing up feelings of fear or insecurity and ask yourself what it is.
- Be honest about what you discover—there's no advantage in lying to yourself.

- Allow yourself to feel your emotions rather than suppressing them.
- Make a plan to deal with what's bothering you.
- Get advice from people you trust, or simply share your dream with them—it helps to talk it through.
- Remember you have the ability to deal with your nightmare in a way that leads to positive results.

## *Faceless Horror = Unknown Fear*

In general, a dream of faceless horror means pretty much what it seems—something is scaring the blazes out of you, but you don't really know what it is. The faceless monster mirrors your unconscious (and therefore unrecognized and unknown) fears about something. It won't be something simple, like having to make a presentation at work or take an exam. It will be a more important issue, one that triggers unconscious fears about survival. You might not be in the untamed wilderness, like our dreamer in Alaska. Just the same, whatever the problem it will feel as if life itself is at risk.

Sometimes a sequence of dreams leading to profound, inner transformation opens with a screaming nightmare featuring faceless horror attacking or pulling you into a dark place. These initiatory nightmares signal the beginning of significant inner change and are the subject for another book. A really horrible nightmare of any kind, especially if it confronts you with overwhelming evil, signals a need to examine your life and consider what changes could be in the wind.

# 11

---

# DEMONS

We have all heard tales of dark creatures with supernatural origins. Age-old myths and stories feature a varied cast of terrible and voracious demons. In the stories the preferred food of demons is usually humans, consumed with glee as their victims scream in agony. It's the original high-protein diet, but not one we want to hear about.

All the great religions of the world feature demons somewhere in their cosmology. They represent the forces of ignorance, negativity, separation from God and unredeemed ego. Demons provide a counterpoint for teachings about divine love, right behavior and redemption. Demons in nightmares take on the characteristics found in the dreamer's cultural and religious upbringing—and more.

The word "nightmare" is in itself a reminder of the fear of demons. In medieval times demons were thought to visit during the night, entertaining themselves by riding the frightened dreamer like a horse—thus "night-mare." They still visit in our dreams and they can still ride us in terror down dark and forbidding roads to a personal dreaming hell. The only difference between us and those terrified dreamers of the Middle Ages is that we know (don't we?) that demons don't really exist.

One peculiar form of human concern has to do with possession. Demonic possession representing ultimate helplessness and degradation has long been a theme of literature, religion and art. In psychopathology there are many cases of people who believe with all their hearts that they are possessed. In the worst cases they act out the destructive commands of their hallucinatory demonic masters, murdering and raping because "the voices told me to." When the line between sanity and serious mental illness is crossed, there is often a demonic figure standing at the border.

Does that mean we are going crazy if we dream of demons? Of course not, but it can certainly feel that way in the dream. If the dreams continue over years they signal a need for professional counseling to resolve the underlying issue. That's true of any really upsetting or disturbing dream that keeps coming back. Demons live in shadow land and represent a powerful, threatening and antagonistic psychological force within. Sometimes a dream of demons can signal the onslaught of change; a demon dream carries the image of erupting shadow content and powerful psychic material. At the least, such dreams indicate there is distress in the unconscious mind and that change may be called for.

The following dreams provide a good example of what I mean.

*For a long time I had dreams that were absolutely terrifying to me. In the deepest of sleep I would be elevated from my bed and would float to the ceiling, sometimes hanging upside down reaching for the floor, trying to get back down. Somehow in my dream I knew I was dreaming and I also knew I was battling with demons and devils. While I was in this struggle, I would get back down to my bed and awaken. I got to the place where I was scared to go to sleep at night. . . .*

Let's stop here for a moment. Does the image of floating above the bed seem familiar to you? It should—it's one of the classic indicators of demonic possession. It was presented dramatically in the movie *The Exorcist.* If you are unfamiliar with the movie, it is a well-known horror film focusing on demonic possession. But this dreamer was a child when her dreams started and had not seen the movie. She was unknowingly tuning in to a description of demonic control that's been around for ages, which the movie used to good advantage. It's unnatural to find yourself floating above the bed, isn't it? A demonic force must be at work to make such a thing happen. Let's follow her story. Eventually her dreams subside, but then pick up again years later when she is an adult.

> . . . *I dreamed I was at the bottom of some steps, looking up with some family members. At the top of the steps was a doorway. I could hear an awful moaning and groaning and a slurring language not known to man. All I could see in the doorway was my sister's feet. She was elevated to the ceiling and the bottom part of her was the only thing visible from where we were standing.*
>
> *My mother and other family members were horrified and upset because we could not get up there and get by her to reach her daughter, my niece. The child was begging us to come and get her because her mother was going to tear her to pieces. . . . I woke up.*
>
> *These horrifying dreams have stuck with me through the years of my childhood and adult life. . . . I often wonder why I have been tortured by these dreams. They are not a drop in the bucket compared to the severity and amount of dreams I have always dreamed. My own family does not like to hear about the dreams I have, because it frightens them so. I don't think I've seen, and they have told me they've never seen, a movie more frightening than what I dream of. Why is this?*

I feel a lot of compassion for this woman, don't you? How would you like to have these awful dreams night after night? If you are one of those who do have frequent demonic dreams, you know exactly how she feels.

## Childhood Abuse and Demon Dreams

Why is this, she asks? Good question, and we can make some assumptions that are probably pretty close to the mark. When people tell me of dreams like this, I usually find they come from an abusive and violent background. As children these folks were sexually and/or physically abused, and they were always psychologically abused. Psychological abuse can be as soul-destroying as anything physical. I often wonder how some parents can be so cruel to their children. I am confronted every day by the consequences, when those children, now adults, come to talk with me.

These dreams are a symptom of severe psychic distress and injury—a wounding of the soul, made visible through nightmares. Her psyche cannot handle the trauma in any rational way. It tries to deal with the injury by presenting terrible nightmares, scenes of emotional and mental distress. Stuck in an unhealed and unresolved loop, the dreams repeat over and over, gnawing at the theme like a dog with a bone.

Her dreams speak of terror and childhood abuse. It's seen in the horrible language, demonic and menacing, the levitation, and especially the child begging for rescue because her mother is going to tear her to pieces. Therapy with a caring and knowledgeable counselor is the best choice for this dreamer. I hope you don't have dreams like this, but if you do it is a good choice for you as well. All of us need a little help and advice from time to time.

Here's another recurring dream about demons.

*. . . The dream always takes place in my bedroom, which makes it seem more real, because when I wake up I am still in the same environment.*

*I am usually in bed when horrible creatures, which identify themselves as the "minion" (I think) grab me by the ankles and pull me up the wall. They laugh at my terror as they hoist me higher and higher. As I get all the way up to the ceiling they disappear, but in the opposite corner of the room I see a swirling black cloud that gets smaller and smaller until it disappears.*

*I have had the same dream for about the last five years, usually once or twice a year.*

Notice any similarities to the other dream? Again the dreamer is lifted against her will, levitated up and away from her bed. She is cut off from earth, cut off from feeling grounded and safe, helplessly dragged to the ceiling while the "minion" laughs. Minion is an interesting word and means a lowly servant, a lackey, an instrument of someone or something—in this case, something evil.

Demon dreams often have this theme of levitation or uncontrolled flight through the air. I think it refers to a sense of helplessness and disconnection. Events in outer life trigger the dream, activating the inner insecurity and fear. It can be hard to pin down exactly, because the original cause may lie buried in the past and not obviously associated with present time. A good example is someone abused as a child who has a demon dream as an adult because she finds herself in a personally confrontational situation. It might or might not be obvious what caused her dream.

This dreamer has the dream whenever things get to be too much for her in waking life. The pressure mounts and then the dream appears. The solution is to find a way to alter outer circumstances and relieve the pressure. She has not been able to do it, thus the reoccurring dream. She doesn't know what is troubling her. The swirling black cloud disappearing into the corner symbolizes a kind of reabsorption. It means the problem has been internalized and isn't going to go away, at least not until she figures out what it is. If you have a reoccurring nightmare, look for something disturbing in your life that needs to be changed and go for it.

The setting of the bedroom is common for demonic dreams. The bedroom is associated with many things—rest, sex and sexuality, illness—in short, anything that we might normally do in bed. Sexual guilt, helplessness, serious illness or significant upset of any kind could be a factor in a demon dream. All the ones I have seen feature a fundamental sense of helplessness. The dreamer is at the mercy of something dramatized by the demonic presence in the dream.

## Dreams of Isolation and Separation

Here's another kind of dream, from a young male dreamer.

*The dream starts off that I'm the only one upstairs, in my bed. It's dark and I can see only a shimmer of light from the living room. Then a howling wind starts to blow and cries out my name. . . . I'm scared; I get out of bed and go to the top of the landing. The wind really picks up and is blowing against me—I have trouble standing straight. The wind howls out my name. . . . I throw myself off the stairs and the wind carries me into the opening of the living room. I'm screaming for help but no one seems to hear me. . . . They carry on watching TV. I'm hanging on to the door opening, but the wind is too strong. I lose my grip, and I'm carried back up to the top of the stairs by the wind, and I see the indentation of a human coming from the ceiling howling my name. . . .*

That's a chiller, isn't it? In this nightmare, the demonic force appears as wind. The dreamer gets out of bed (we're back in the bedroom again), is overwhelmed by the wind, and is carried back and forth. He can't get help—no one hears him. He's separated from the people watching TV in the living room, which are symbols of normalcy and his waking life—where he lives. Something awful is coming out of the ceiling at him, while the wind howls his name . . . brrrr!

This is a dream driven by inner feelings of separation and isolation. We see again the familiar image of lifting away from the earth, from the basis of being, from the grounding aspect, from everything that makes him (and us) feel connected and safe in a universe where there is order and predictability. The image of people watching TV provides a clue that the theme is separation and isolation, since they ignore his cries for help. Isolated within himself (it's his dream), he feels alienated in the real, waking world.

Our dreamer is alone, at the mercy of the howling wind. When a howling wind calls your name in a dream, you'd better listen! His mind is attempting to help him, even though it may not feel like that in the dream. Something is trying to emerge into his awareness (the image on the ceiling) but he is not able to see and accept it. The conflict is causing the dream. It isn't something he really wants to know about on a conscious level, probably because it is deeply disturbing or upsetting. We are all very good at denying things we don't want to see or know about in our lives, but our nightmares will not let us off easily if it's really important.

In earlier times people had no way to understand the truth about demonic dreams. They thought the dreams were actual visitations by the minions of hell (there's that word again). Demon dreams contributed to the cosmology of demonic forces, described according to their characteristics. In Western Europe one particularly heinous demon was called a succubus. The succubus was a female demon who visited in the night, bringing terror and a kind of horrible sexuality to her unfortunate male victims. Here is an example of this kind of dream, but it doesn't come from centuries ago—it was dreamed recently. The medieval succubus is alive and well, at least in our nightmares.

*It was nearly 5 A.M., and I was wondering if I should grab my pistol and check out the house. My dream scared me so bad. . . . I felt a crushing, evil, female presence on top of my chest, like someone had buried both knees into me. I struggled to breathe.*

*The woman told me to let my girlfriend die, as if we had been discussing her for some time. When she spoke it was in a low, demonic voice and pain ripped through my body. Then I woke up and I swear I heard her voice one last time, even being awake. For some reason I was so short on breath I was about to pass out. I then yelled, "Oh God, don't let me die!" I stood up, and my legs were extremely wobbly because all of my extremities were asleep. I guess from the time it took me to get the blood flowing in my arms and legs they had been asleep for a while. . . .*

## *Demon Dreams and Physical Illness*

These are serious dreams, not least because of the bodily effects the dreamer is describing. This kind of dream must never be ignored. It could signal much more than underlying emotional issues (like problems in relationship with a girlfriend). The physical effects demand that he see a doctor for a checkup. The symptoms he describes could be consistent with a mild heart attack, for example. A message of poor health might appear in his dream as a demon saying his girlfriend must die. Girlfriend = romance = heart. See how it comes together? We look at the association of images and thoughts. If this interpretation is correct, the dream is warning him of danger because of a heart problem. Poor circulation when he wakes up is another clue pointing in this direction.

Many ailments can produce a nightmare of being unable to breathe. Sometimes our body signals come across in our dreams. We dream of a bathroom toilet and wake needing to relieve ourselves. We suffer from apnea (a sleep disorder that interferes with normal breathing) and we dream of suffocation. We dream of snow and ice and wake to find the blankets on the floor. We have a heart problem and dream of a demon with her knees in our chest. Even so, all of the images can still be seen as conveying a broader meaning.

The demonic female presence in the dream above is a signal of something very wrong for this dreamer. She may not be a demon in reality, but the consequences of ignoring the dream might be just as destructive as if she were truly an emissary from Satan.

## IF YOU DREAM OF DEMONS

- Look closely at your life and identify anything that makes you feel powerless and helpless. If you find something, do whatever you can to change the situation.
- Ask yourself if you are feeling "cut off" from things, from peo-

ple and friends. If you are feeling depressed, isolated and alone, without the resources you need to nurture and sustain yourself, you may see Satan's minions in your dreams.

- Be realistic about how the dreams are affecting you. If you have ongoing, terrifying dreams of demons that destroy sleep and leave you feeling exhausted in the morning, consider seeking professional help to deal with the underlying issues.

- Remember that nightmares are an urgent message from the unconscious to the waking mind. What are the terrifying dreams trying to tell you? Even if you don't really know the specifics, you can probably get a general idea by simply taking a look at your current life situation and identifying problem areas.

- Be honest when you ask yourself what the problem might be. The only person you deceive by falling short in the honesty department is yourself.

- Remember you have the ability to understand the underlying issues, whatever they may be, and deal successfully with them. Within each one of us lies the solution to our particular problem.

# 12

---

# CHOKING, DROWNING, AND SUFFOCATION

Choking and suffocation dreams are about relationship with life. Choking cuts off the breath, and breath, like blood, is essential to life. When we lose passion for life, or when we feel oppressed and invalidated by what is happening in our life, we might have a suffocation dream.

We have lots of ways of expressing frustration with life that use metaphors of suffocation, choking or drowning. We say, "I feel suffocated by my work," or, "He choked" (meaning he froze up in the midst of something, lost the flow), or "I felt like I was drowning," meaning the speaker felt completely overwhelmed. Our nightmares use the same themes, much more graphically, to convey the same ideas of being overwhelmed and losing our sense of self.

This particular theme seems fairly popular in Nightmare Land, and often the dreamer will find the dream repeating regularly. I can't tell you how many times people come to me with a repeating nightmare. As you've seen in the earlier chapters, it's very common. It always means the same thing, in a general way: the dreamer is not getting the message. It's like the saying, "Those who don't learn from history are doomed to repeat it." If we don't understand what our nightmare is trying to tell us, we are very likely doomed to repeat it until we do.

> . . . Since the death of my father I've had a terrifying dream. In the dream there are always different things happening. Sometimes I'm alone watching TV, sometimes I'm at a party with a bunch of people or friends, and sometimes I'm out eating. The dream always ends with me choking. I'm choking on my own teeth, an ice cube, a hot dog. . . . It's always the same feeling. Even after I wake up I'm choking for a while. I have this dream at least three times a month. . . .

Here it's the theme of choking that repeats, not the exact dream sequence. She always ends up choking. What are these nightmares trying to tell her? It helps to know a little about the dreamer, who was very close to her parents. Her father is dead; her mother is in a nursing home. She feels guilty because she doesn't visit her mother as often as she thinks she should. She's the kind of person people turn to when something is bothering them, dumping their emotional problems on her sympathetic ear and seeking her advice. But whom does she turn to?

The answer is nobody, now that her mother is incapacitated and her father is gone. She bottles it up inside. She never complains. But something inside of her has had enough. Do you think this might explain her dreams of choking?

Her unconscious mind wants her to express herself and let go of the pent up feelings she carries. She needs to dump on someone else for a change. She still grieves for her father. No one can hurry grieving, but it's a lot worse and it takes longer to get through if we try to carry it alone, inside ourselves. These nightmares are trying to make a point: until she does something about it she will continue to have them.

The things that choke her are all symbolic of nourishment. Her teeth, for example: we chew food with teeth, and teeth often refer to issues of self-empowerment and nourishment. The ice cubes from drinks are part of partying and engagement with life, part of nourishing oneself. A hot dog: food again. She is feeling unnur-tured, unnourished and guilty. The feelings are choking her, cut-ting her off from life.

The kinds of things that choke us in a dream offer a clue to the nature of the underlying problem. In the dream above it is a need to nourish and take care of herself. In the next dream it is similar but different.

*Over the past few months I've had the same dream. Sometimes I can go for months and not have it and then other times I dream it constantly.*

*In the dream I am choking. I always swallow something (the item is always different, with examples being a ring, perfume, pens), and then I wake up distressed and coughing until I realize that it is only a dream.*

In this nightmare the things choking her aren't food but they stand for something that nurtures (or not) just the same. Perfume, for example, is usually associated with feminine things. Some of the colognes and such that some men wear are really perfume in disguise, but it's still generally seen as feminine, not masculine. Pens and perfume—perhaps she's burning out on the job or over-riding a desire to express herself in more feminine ways. Pens are usually associated with mental things like writing things down, although we might ask if the pen is a symbol for self-expression. It would depend on what she feels about the image.

Whatever the cause, consciously taking care of herself in some new and different way is part of the solution. It always is when choking dreams begin, unless there is a medical reason triggering the sensation of choking in the dream. If it's medical, chances are you already know you have a problem with breathing. If it's not medical, something is choking the life out of you in a very real sense, whether it's a dead-end job, a failing relationship or just plain frustration with life.

*I was sitting in the woods by the water with a friend of mine. The water was not clean and I wanted to go, but the only way to go was to climb a tree. We climbed all the way to the top and I noticed that my friend was not in clothing, just wearing underwear now. That didn't seem important to me. . . . I told him to be careful, because the tree was older than when the Pilgrims were here.*

*I climbed back down halfway and then jumped down and asked my friend to hand me my purse. He dropped it down and it rolled down the hill, plunging into the water. I then ran down and jumped in after it. I had to swim under a cement wall to get it.*

*The way down and getting it was easy. I clutched it in my hand and turned back. To my dismay I found it a lot harder to swim back. As I got closer I felt like my lungs were going to explode, so I tried to swim up but I didn't quite make it. I began to die underwater and I woke up gasping for breath.*

There are really three parts to this dream: by looking at each we can figure out the meaning in a broad sense. In part one she and her friend climb the tree that is "older than when the Pilgrims were here." That is dream talk for a long-standing issue that has her "treed." She's near unclean water and wants to go but can only escape by climbing the tree. The water represents the unknown problem. The boyfriend loses his clothes because something she normally does in a masculine way (read structured, organized, logical, mental) needs to be revealed. It is part of the unknown problem.

In the next scene she gets down out of the tree and asks for her purse, but it lands in the water. What does the purse represent? A woman's purse is many things—more than a man's wallet, but similar in an important way. It contains many symbols of one's life. Money (nourishment); credit cards; identification papers of various kinds, like a driver's license (ability to get around, empowerment); address book; cosmetics (presentation of self in the world); and so on. A purse is a very good dream image for one's identity in the world, of a combination of things reflecting something about the owner. Because so much of the dream involves the purse, the theme is her sense of self, her sense of who she is. Something unseen (the unclean water that bothers her) is threatening her sense of identity.

OK so far? I'm walking you through this fairly complicated dream so you can get a better sense of how it's done. We look at each event or symbolic image and then make associations with them. That will give us a good hit on the dream. You can do the same thing with your choking nightmare.

She dives into the water, swims under a barrier and grabs the purse. So far, so good. This part of the dream says she actually does have the inner resources to get past the obstacles for understanding, whatever they are—that's the meaning of swimming under the barrier. But there's trouble getting back to the surface. She is drowning and wakes gasping for breath. This is a pretty clear reference to difficulty she has in understanding what is going wrong for her in her life, what exactly is threatening her sense of self. It's still under the surface, just like in the dream.

If this were my dream I would make an assumption I was feeling unconsciously threatened by some situation in my life. Once I figured out what it was, I'd try to do something about it. "Unconscious" simply means we don't know what something is, it's not in our awareness. We often know a lot of things before they appear in our waking awareness, and our dreams, especially nightmares, can give us an early heads-up.

## IF YOU DREAM OF CHOKING

If you have a nightmare about suffocating, choking or drowning, ask yourself these questions:

- Is something going on in my life that feels oppressive or confining to me?
- Do I have a medical condition (like asthma, emphysema or apnea) that might contribute to my dream?
- Am I feeling trapped about something and unable to change it?
- Are circumstances in my life making me feel panicked and unable to cope?
- Am I out of my depth and overwhelmed by my life right now?

Answering yes to any of these might explain why you are having the dream. Take a gentle look at what's happening in your life, don't panic, and realize you can take steps that will lead you to a better situation.

# 13

## TEETH

Teeth—what would we do without them? Possibly the most common nightmare of all is one where we dream about our teeth falling out. This is just a short chapter, but I felt it needed its own place because so many of us have this kind of dream.

A dream of losing teeth or feeling them crumble, crack and fall to the floor in a bloody mess is particularly disturbing. We remember dreams like this. On my Web site dream board, dreams of teeth in trouble are very common. Unfortunately many so-called dream books give very inaccurate interpretations of this symbol. This can lead to considerable stress and worry when none is called for. Here's an example, taken from the dream board, which illustrates perfectly what I mean.

*. . . I'm a twenty-seven-year-old female, working as a computer programmer and just starting my Ph.D. in computer science. I'm married, no children, and living here in New York far away from my family.*

*I had this strange and freaky dream yesterday. I was in a room with my mom and dad and suddenly my upper-front tooth fell out on the ground (it looked huge). The other front tooth became very loose, about to fall out. My dad saw it and tried to pull it out. I freaked and ran into another room and closed the door.*

*My mom has a book about dream interpretation. The book says "losing teeth" means losing a member of your family, i.e., someone will die. Upper teeth symbolize someone older than you, i.e., parents, grandparents, aunt, etc. Lower teeth symbolize someone younger.*

*I'm so concerned and worried. I really don't want to believe what the book says. . . .*

I wouldn't want to believe it either. That is complete nonsense, and it's the kind of thing that makes people think dream interpretation is a waste of time. Like many "traditional" interpretations, it is based on folklore and superstition. This particular interpretation of losing teeth has its roots in ancient China. You can rest easy out there; losing teeth in a dream has nothing at all to do with someone close to you dying. What it has to do with is some inner concern, symbolized by the teeth.

Teeth are used to speak and communicate, to chew food, to protect and attack (in more primitive times), to convey feelings (a big smile or a tight-lipped expression), and have cosmetic value in a world where good looks are valued highly. All of these uses can be referred to in a dream where our teeth end up on the floor or swallowed, like the dream in the last chapter.

Having a hard time at work and feeling disempowered by your boss? Maybe you will dream about your teeth falling out. Can't get your point of view across in the world and feeling frustrated because no one seems to value what you say? Teeth on the floor are a good possibility in your dreams. Can't seem to get control of your life so that you feel reasonably nourished by it? Another good reason to dream about teeth.

*I have had many dreams where as I'm talking my teeth are breaking and crumbling in my mouth. I have to keep spitting them out as it happens. Or I dream my teeth are loose and wobbling, I am stressing about losing them, and they usually end up coming out. . . .*

This nightmare is about not getting heard and acknowledged. Imagine a scene in real life where someone begins talking and then starts spitting out teeth! If she were eating in the dream the meaning might shift in the direction of what does or doesn't nurture her, but here she is talking when the teeth start to crumble. It's an issue of self-expression for this dreamer. She needs to seek out ways to express herself and get acknowledged for it.

*All of my back teeth are falling out. It's an awful feeling. . . .*

I suppose that dream book with all the good ideas about teeth and family and relatives dying might say the back teeth falling out means your pet dog is in danger, but we know better, don't we? This is more in the nourishment area. The back teeth are right before the throat, right before we swallow. Take out your back teeth and eating becomes a lot harder. The muscles that work the jaw and the back teeth in chewing are very powerful. So this could also be a dream about feeling a lack of power.

I hope you are beginning to understand how to look at nightmares. If you dream about your teeth falling out, don't rush to your dentist (unless you are having dental problems).

## When Your Teeth Fall Out in Dreams

- Ask yourself if you feel frustrated about the way people listen to you. Perhaps you need to improve your communication skills.
- Notice if you are having trouble communicating something important. The frustration may be giving you nightmares.
- Do you feel at the mercy of other people and events? If so, make an effort to change your situation so you feel more in control.
- If you have the dream more than once, try to identify a pattern of similar external situations that might provide a stimulus for the dream. For example, perhaps you are not comfortable with speaking in public, or making presentations at work. These can be situations that set the stage for a toothless sleep experience.

- If you have actual dental problems, stop postponing that trip to the dentist. The dream could be telling you that the health of your mouth needs attention.

# 14

# FANGS AND CLAWS

Most of us like animals. We have pets we care for, companions to help us through life. There are animals that work for us, animals that entertain us, animals that amuse us and animals that frighten us. Animals are so much a part of life that it makes sense they would show up in our dreams. Dream animals can take on a lot of different meanings. Native American and worldwide shamanic spiritual traditions see animals as powerful guardians or allies, showing up in dreams or visions to teach us or aid us. There are also animal enemies in those traditions, and there can be animal enemies in our nightmares as well. We aren't going to look at the shamanic teachings about dream animals here, but if you are interested there are many books available to help you learn more.

Frequently nightmares with animals end up with the dreamer torn to pieces or eaten alive. Sometimes we fight and kill the attacking critter but feel guilty when we wake up. That is particularly true for people who "wouldn't hurt a fly," or vegetarians who sometimes find themselves slaughtering menacing cows from hell in their dreams. Whatever our outer ideas about animals may be, in the world of nightmares all bets are off. If cute and cuddly Fluffy the cat tries to tear your throat out in your dream, it doesn't mean Fluffy is really out to get you in real life. But the symbol of Fluffy is important, chosen by your dreaming mind to tell you something.

The setting of a dream always gives us information. Here's a nightmare set among friends; perhaps the dream is making a comment about them.

*I have this dream where I am in a house with a lot (like twenty) of my friends and get chased by a tiger they say is friendly. Since it's their pet, they won't hurt it. It chases me and then bites me, but I get away and try to hide. Of course there's no place to hide. Right before it eats me I wake up.*

At least he woke up before the tiger actually ate him! This is a young male dreamer. The tiger belongs to his friends; they won't help, and he's threatened. Do you think the dream is trying to tell him something about his friends; or at least about his relationship to them? On one level, that could be true. Perhaps he needs to rethink what friendship is about or what these friends really mean to him.

A more likely meaning, and the next level of interpretation, is that the dream is not about real people but is addressing inner insecurities. It's tough for adolescents to learn how people socialize and get along—the rules change frequently and it's a little frightening out there. There's a huge amount of peer pressure to conform to the particular customs of the teen subculture. The culture can be quite cruel, even merciless, to someone who doesn't fit in. I think this dream reflects that reality. It's pointing out unspoken insecurity and fear of falling out of favor.

*I was surrounded by white wolves that began to be playfully aggressive with me. I began to feel concerned as I realized the strength they were beginning to force on me. When I realized it, it was too late and they proceeded to kill me.*

Unlike our first example, this adult male dreamer didn't wake up in time to escape death. That's significant. When you die in a dream something is ending or completing, undergoing a funda-mental shift. It can also be a warning to the outer mind that some-thing is getting ready to change in a big way.

Wolves are intriguing animals, intelligent and dangerous, asso-ciated with freedom and primal instinct. They are romanticized or vilified according to our particular point of view. In today's society wolves have a powerful collective meaning, making them effective dream symbols. How you think about wolves will be reflected in the dream. But how you think about wolves in real life may lead you into a different experience than expected when the wolves show up in your dream.

This dreamer likes wolves in real life. The dream begins with the wolves appearing playfully aggressive, not really dangerous. It's only after they become more intense that he realizes he's in trouble, and then they kill him. It's a dream of suppressed urges, thoughts and ideas not acceptable to him in waking life.

We all repress primal urges—it's part of being civilized, part of being accepted into the human social community. Primal means basic and instinctual in this sense. The dreamer is like the rest of us. He's learned to abide by the rules of civilized behavior. But sometimes in the name of civilization we go too far, shutting down primal levels at the expense of expressing ourselves in vibrant and energizing ways that give meaning to our lives.

The wolves in his nightmare are white. White stands for puri-ty, cleansing, innocence and especially "not black." Black is often a reference (in dreams) to shadow forces at work, things hidden from the conscious mind. In this dream white is a symbol for whit-ing out the black, whitewashing, covering over something in essence wolf-like, primal and basic, not innocent or pure accord-ing to the idealized judgments of his outer mind. The playful white wolves end up killing him. They symbolize repression of primal and instinctual forces. The dream is a warning, telling the dreamer efforts to suppress his instinctual nature will lead to a dangerous situation.

He is also warned that he can't play with what the wolves rep-resent—he has to respect their power and treat it with caution. He needs to strike a balance and find a way to express some of this "wolf" energy; if he doesn't there could be consequences. In my experience the consequences of ignoring dream warnings range from mild depression to serious illness. I don't know what that balance might look like for him. I do know it means doing something that reanimates him and gives him a new sense of intensity in life.

*I've had this dream recently. . . . I was walking down a long flight of slippery stairs. At the bottom of the stairs were several large, snarling dogs. I couldn't get back up the stairs, because they were too slippery, and I fell to the ground.*

*I got up and ran, with the dogs chasing me. I ran through a dark forest surrounded in fog, with the dogs still snarling at my heels, until I came to a clearing and ran into a junkyard. The dogs refused to follow me into the junkyard but paced around the perimeter, still snarling and barking. Suddenly I heard strange clicking noises. When I looked down, ugly insects came up from the ground and started to crawl on me. I woke up terrified.*

*I also had a snarling dog dream several years ago. I was lost in the mountains with my daughter (who was about seven at the time) when we encountered snarling dogs. They didn't attack us but kept threatening to. I took her by the hand, stepped over a mountain ledge and walked down into a valley with her away from the dogs. They did not follow but kept barking and snarling.*

It's interesting that this woman had a snarling-dog nightmare in the past. Notice she still recalls it, years later—that is typical of powerful nightmares. Unlike most dreams, which fade quicker than thought with the morning light, nightmares may be remembered for all of our lives.

At the root of this dream is a problem that's been around at least since she had the first dream, and the bad news is that it's getting worse. There is more urgency in the second dream, more terror and more impact. There are many clues in both dreams to give us a general idea of the meaning.

In the first dream the most important image, aside from the

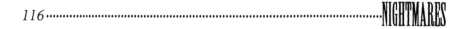

dogs, is the daughter. When we see a person we know in our dreams, even a family member or a child, the figure is still a symbol. That's easy to forget. Most of the time we think the dream has something to do with the real person. It does, but only in the sense that the actual person has certain qualities used by the dreaming mind to get a point across. In this case the daughter mirrors the dreamer herself, a reference to something needing protection.

The dogs are graphic symbols of feeling threatened and at risk. That is also true in the second dream, but there's a difference and it's not a good one. The second dream begins with a descent down slippery stairs. That's a sure giveaway we are looking at a dream of the shadow. Down the slippery steps is a dream metaphor for going down into the depths of the unconscious mind. She doesn't really know what the problem is in her waking mind, but something in her knows there's a problem and it wants relief.

The chase through the forest in the fog reminds me of the Sherlock Holmes adventure called "The Hound of the Baskervilles." In that classic a devilish glowing dog roams the foggy moors at night, scaring the blazes out of everyone, providing a suitably gothic touch to the Victorian tale. Fog is another reference to the fact she can't clearly see what is going on. She's "in a fog" about it. OK so far?

The dogs halt outside the junkyard, but keep watch on the perimeter. She's trapped. And then it really gets horrible, as ugly insects emerge from the junkyard ground and begin to crawl on her. Doesn't it make *your* skin crawl?

The junkyard represents stored-up junk. "Junk" is dreamspeak for old fears, angers, hurts, emotional injuries, frustrations and self-judgmental ideas we all carry around with us. The horrible insects emerging from the junkyard ground add emphasis and suggest the issues are very old, very basic and very disturbing. It could be childhood wounds coming back to haunt her, or it could be something else. My bet would go towards childhood, but I admit to a certain bias in that direction. That's because I see so many people in my practice who are struggling as adults with crippling psychological wounds incurred in childhood.

Here are two powerful dreams from one woman, revealing sadness and inner loss.

*Before my divorce, my husband, my children and I had moved back to our home state from Montana. On the night before my husband left, I had a nightmare. I never have them. This one night I awoke and there beside my bed was the most evil-looking dog I have ever seen, like the ones in* Ghostbusters, *yet more terrifying; I was way beyond the word "terrified," I could only tremble and cry. I guess I was trying to scream in my sleep when my spouse at the time said, "It's OK."*

*That was the end of it and I never saw the dog creature again until last week. My best friend in Montana committed suicide two years ago. It devastated all of us; this was something none of us were prepared for. Last week the dog came back and this time my fear was greater. It was like seeing hell from the front door. It was misty. In the mist came my friend, her face so, so sad. All she said was, "Beware of being misled and believe in God. Listen, listen, listen. I can never come back and I can never be your friend."*

*I wanted to reach out for her; it was as though she felt every pain there ever was, yet I knew if I tried to reach her the dog would devour me. It terrified me. I don't understand this and it does scare me.*

Whew! That's heavy—what a disturbing dream. Have you seen the movie *Ghostbusters*? It's a comedy, but has powerful horror images that come straight out of our collective unconscious, including the evil dogs. They are not cute puppies you would like to meet, but guardians of a gateway into hell.

What do you think that dog symbolizes? We can take it for granted it is overwhelming fear about something. Like other kinds of demons, the dog cannot be controlled or overcome. It represents the essence of vulnerability. The first appearance of the demon dog is on the night before her first husband leaves her. I don't think that's a coincidence, do you?

Let's jump to the second dream. Even though it appears to be very different, it is still addressing the same issue: grief and loss the dreamer feels. In the first dream it's triggered by the end of her marriage; in the second it's triggered by something else in her life and takes on the image of her dead friend. In both dreams the underlying issue is about emotional loss that still hurts, even though the events are in the past. The second dream is also trying to warn her about something. That is shown by the message from the friend.

"Beware of being misled. . . ." sounds like a message to me! Something is going on in this woman's life that has not yet emerged in her awareness. Or perhaps she is in denial—either way, she is told to take notice. The reference to believing in God reflects ideas about God as a source of nourishment and protection. It's a reminder to keep emotionally centered.

"I can never come back and be your friend . . ." is harder to understand at first. Some might see it as a direct statement from beyond the grave—after all, the friend committed suicide, a damning sin in many religions. But it is not a direct message from the dead; it's a message from the inner self. The dead friend represents all of the loss and grief in her life—core issues that have been around a long time. By making the dream image say these words, the unconscious emphasizes the depth of sadness she feels and reflects it back to her waking mind. The dreaming mind is giving her a status report—it's not providing any solutions.

True understanding of any dream involves jumping into the implication of the dream message. In this case, the implication is (1) something is up in her outer life that must be looked at and understood ("don't be misled") and (2) she is feeling saddened and upset about something.

I think the problem is related to feeling unloved and unwanted, starting early on and reinforced by later life and experience (like her divorce). She would like to heal this feeling—who wouldn't? But she is terrified to deal with the issue, since it would mean confronting negative ideas about herself and stirring up painful feelings. You can see how nightmare interpretation can get tricky and sometimes very sensitive.

## KEY QUESTIONS

If you dream of animals attacking, you can ask yourself a few key questions to help determine the meaning of the dream:

- What kind of animal is it? The type of animal carries a symbolic meaning. For example, wolves are different from horses and we have different ideas about them as animals.
- What is your idea about the animal?
- What is the setting of the dream? By looking at the setting you might get a good idea of where the problem is focused—like the junkyard in the dream given earlier that symbolized old issues.
- How do you feel about expressing emotions? Perhaps the dream is trying to point out a need to express yourself in ways you might normally avoid. Anger, for example, might not be an emotion you think is acceptable.
- Are you fooling yourself about something? That could be the case when you see the dream animal as normally friendly and nonthreatening in outer life. In other words, things are not as they appear to be.

Try these questions out and see how they fit. In any case, go easy on yourself and allow your intuition to point the way.

# 15

## THE END OF THE WORLD

People have been dreaming about the end of the world for a long time. I don't need to tell you about the many religious and secular prophecies describing the end of all life as we know it. From television fantasies of alien doom to medical pronouncements predicting worldwide plague, fear of final disaster is alive and well. Our culture is chock-full of images of death and destruction. Is it any wonder our nightmares might also present these same images in our worst dreams?

I was brought up during the height of the cold war, when there was a real possibility we might all be incinerated in a radioactive cloud. Of course all of us kids were told we were safe—all we had to do was get under our desks when the alarm sounded and everything would turn out fine. Uh-huh. Years later, as a young adult in New York City, I woke one night in a state of complete terror and panic, convinced an H-bomb had just dropped. I thought I was in my last second of mortal awareness. A siren passing in the hot summer night outside my open apartment window triggered the dream.

My dreaming mind picked the bomb as an inner image of the intense stress I felt at the time. End of the world dreams are a perfect way to announce we are reaching a point of stress that is intolerable. The theme can be war, natural disaster, plague or alien invasion—it doesn't matter. What matters is that the world ends in our dreams, at least the world as we know it.

## Dreams of War and The Bomb

*I am back living at my parents' house and I look out the kitchen window. I see all sorts of army vehicles and soldiers passing by on the gravel road. I run outside to the front yard, looking toward the town, and I notice warplanes flying above. I feel our country is under attack by another country. Then I look toward the town again and I see the end of the world—a mushroom cloud appears where once was my town. My life flashes before me, and I have this helpless, gut feeling that I am going to die.*

I wonder if there is a better symbol of helplessness and mortal fear than the mushroom cloud? By now there are probably few people in the world who have not been exposed to this terrible image of unchecked doom and destruction: all-consuming, all-destroying, a hellish and colossal cloud roiling into the sky, signaling the inexorable end of life.

When the mushroom cloud appears in your nightmare, it's saying you are feeling vulnerable and threatened. It is also telling you change is on the way, possibly of life-altering magnitude. Our sense of identity and self, our ego, does not like big changes. I would go so far as to say our egos hate most important change, even if we have initiated it. A nuclear bomb exploding in your dreams is a statement about the ego's fear of what may be coming. To the ego it *is* the end of the world.

The dream above is a dream of insecurity. The dreamer is back at his parents' house—a major clue, telling us his nightmare is really about feeling unable to cope as an adult. He has returned to his parents, meaning he has retreated to an earlier stage of development when he didn't have the capabilities, or the responsibilities, of an adult. His parents' house also symbolizes a context of earlier learning and experience, suggesting he may be caught up in some childhood pattern keeping him from resolving the problem. Whatever is stressing him out, he feels unable to cope with it. It feels like the end to him. He needs to identify the problem and take steps to resolve it.

Sometimes people are afraid these kinds of dreams are prophetic, foretelling an actual nuclear attack. We still live with the possibility of nuclear war. No one can think this would lead to anything except the most terrible consequences, the end of the world in every way that matters. In nightmares, though, it is our internal fears rising as an atomic cloud, not a foreshadowing of war.

*I am always dreaming of war, either the impending detonation of a nuclear weapon over my city or a slow-moving missile on a course for me or those close to me. In the dreams I normally have prior knowledge of impact . . . a feeling of menace and doom prevails while I wait for the blast.*

*I always survive the blast. Usually I'm trying to warn others and worrying about my family. I fall to the ground or hide in a ditch to protect myself. . . . I have had dreams that come true and wish these ones would leave me.*

The woman who had this dream lives in an unusually peaceful part of the world, a pleasant place to live, not likely to be at the top of target lists for nuclear attack. Even so, I'd be nervous, too, if I had a history of dreams coming true in other areas. But this isn't a dream of impending attack in a literal sense. It's another example of a nightmare highlighting inner insecurity

Because she says she "always" has these dreams of war and destruction, it's safe to assume some regular context or situation in her outer life brings up concerns for her well-being and the people she cares for. Family in a dream is usually about our inner "family," not the real people. In other words, her fears are for herself. Only she can identify what the problem is; only she has the power to challenge it. When she does, the skies of her dreams will no longer be filled with missiles and bombs.

*I have had these dreams almost every night for the past eighteen years . . . The world has almost come to an end. Everywhere I go there are the remains of people, buildings and things, burned, bombed and destroyed. The sun does not shine and the remaining people who survive are desperate for anything they can steal or eat. They rape anyone they can. They are like mindless robots, foaming at the mouth for anything.*

*I am always running from these people and saving and defending the few good people left. I lead them to safety. I am their leader, and when they refuse to listen to me they die at the hands of their own foolishness. I never die, they chase me and come close to capture, but I always escape, fight and kill them.*

*I live in a big mansion on the top of a hill. It has been burned and bombed and once belonged to someone else, but I have taken it over and made it my home. It is gigantic and mysterious, no furniture or any nice things. I live like an animal, sleeping on edge, because it is kill or be killed.*

This nightmare signals the need for outside guidance to get to the root of things, especially since it has been going on for so long. I don't know the dreamer—this dream comes from the Web site. If I were working with her, I would want to know about her background and her life, because the dream indicates a lot of internal conflict.

She lives in a burned-out mansion on the top of a hill, a mansion that once belonged to someone else. But it's her dream, and that house on the hill has always belonged to her—there's no one else inside, dreaming for her. By presenting an image of a destroyed mansion with no nice things to ease and comfort her, the dreaming mind is trying to make a point. What do you think a burned-out mansion could mean?

If you guessed the dream is trying to get her to see that she feels abandoned and forced to rely on her own resources for love, life and nourishment, you would be right. The mansion on a hill represents security, prosperity and nourishment. Many of us have a vision tucked away somewhere of a mansion on a hill, a kind of culmination of life's best results and desires made real. But her mansion is destroyed; it is a symbol for exactly the opposite of all those good things. In her dream that's where she lives, a hostile and unforgiving landscape lacking comfort and safety. I have a lot of compassion for her, because I know things can't be easy or pleasant for her in waking life.

Lots of people dream of attack by the armies of an evil invader. Whom you see as the enemy depends on where you come from. Many Americans dream of Nazi armies or Russian troops, but if you come from somewhere else it could just as easily be American soldiers coming after you in your dreams. Big armies of dream enemies represent an overwhelming force that can't be dealt with. You can fight, you can run and hide, but you can't defeat them. These armies always seem completely destructive. They rape, murder, loot, burn and destroy anything and everything in their way.

When armies of enemies appear in your dreams, something is really getting to you. They are a message of feeling helpless and powerless. Helplessness and powerlessness appear in many different kinds of nightmares—it is probably the underlying feeling in most of them.

Here are some broad interpretations of common end-of-the-world dream symbols. Look at your dream and then try to get beyond your usual ideas about what something means. For example, if you are a religious person and you dream of Armageddon, you might get caught in thinking the dream was actually prophesying the coming of the last days. Chances are that's not the case, so your challenge is to understand what is making you feel threatened and, perhaps, afraid.

## COMMON END-OF-THE-WORLD SYMBOLS

**Tidal waves.** Tidal waves are often about emotional issues, feelings that need expression or a sense of something coming that can disrupt your life dramatically. One of the many symbolic meanings for water is emotion. An ocean of water can represent all of our unconscious desires, unexpressed thoughts and more. A tidal wave arises out of that great expanse of our inner self and threatens to wash us away.

**Earthquakes.** Earthquakes shake the ground we stand on. It's not necessary to have actually felt an earthquake in real life to get a 9.0 on the Richter scale in your dreams. Dream earthquakes encompass all of the usual suspects: fear, insecurity, destruction, overwhelming helplessness and terror. A dream earthquake may suggest something more immediate than a tidal wave. While a tidal wave can represent the kind of emotional issues we all keep bottled up inside, an earthquake may refer to something that has shaken us in waking life, disturbing our fundamental way of seeing things. Our foundation is shaken.

**Tornadoes.** Tornadoes are a very popular dream image. Sometimes they can be health-related, but mostly they seem to signal upheaval of some sort approaching. By upheaval, I don't mean a real tornado. I mean an inner upheaval, a "twister" of the inner self, foreshadowing emotional turbulence.

**Lightning.** Being struck by lightning is a powerful dream image. You might not like it, but it signals irreversible change taking place. That doesn't mean your whole life is going to turn upside down! What it means is that something has been initiated within your unconscious, something has begun. It's a jolt of pure energy, electrifying and transforming. If you are hit by lightning in your dream, or a bolt of lightning lands nearby, it's a sign from your inner self that things are moving within and going to change.

**Big storms.** Big storms are a little like tidal waves or armies. They represent an overwhelming force that must be reckoned with. Sometimes we might have a dream foreshadowing a coming emotional storm: dark clouds building on the dream horizon, a nightmare weatherman telling us a storm is approaching. Whatever the nature of the inner problem, forewarned is forearmed. If you know something's coming you might be able to take steps to head it off or express things differently.

**Fire.** Fire is always important in any dream. Fire means transformation. It's up to you to discover exactly what it means for you. Do you need to make a dramatic shift in your life? Do you need to let go of something or challenge your ideas about it? Whatever the dream is trying to tell you, one thing is sure: something old is passing and something new will enter to take its place. Fire transforms completely, changing the form of whatever it touches. Sometimes you can get a sense of what is changing by looking at what is burning in the dream. Is the city (or a building) burning? Then structure, ideas and ways of seeing things are in for review. Is the forest burning? You are looking at something more instinctual, more natural and more primal. Here, too, something is about to change.

**Invasion by enemy forces.** As you saw in examples above, invading armies signal a growing sense of helplessness and confusion about something. It's overwhelm time. Perhaps you have too much work, too many problems, too much stress. The solution is to reduce stress levels in your life, try to make conscious choices about the things getting to you, and change the situation until stress is reduced.

**Alien invasions from outer space.** This is a variation on the invading army theme. The difference is that aliens represent something basically unfamiliar and foreign (alien) to your waking mind. That means you may have to do some fancy guesswork to arrive at the meaning. A foreign army invading still has human form, so although it may be foreign to the waking consciousness it at least has some common element of familiarity. It can be identified. But aliens fall outside the realm of common human experience. Alien invasion means you are dealing with something you would not normally be thinking about.

**Nuclear attack.** Some dreams present us with a surprise attack. In that case, our dreaming mind is trying to warn us of impending emotional surprise. Some dreams give warning of the attack. We are still faced with the results, but have some capability to prepare, some knowledge of what is presented in the dream if we but look for it. In either case, we face some kind of upheaval or are feeling strongly at the effect of something unpleasant. These dreams are a little like fire dreams, because they represent destruction of old form. The difference may be in the extent of the change, represented by the extent of the damage in the dream.

**Missile attack.** A variation of the nuclear attack theme, since the missiles are usually nuclear in the dream. Ballistic missiles are one of the nasty variations on annihilation humans have created. If possible, we are more vulnerable to missile attacks than to conventional bombing. It's the preferred choice in modern warfare for cost-efficient and devastating destruction. We all know, because we have been told time and time again, that missiles are almost impossible to stop. You can see they make a perfect dream symbol for feeling helpless and at the mercy of external forces. At the risk of raising the ghost of Sigmund Freud, there could be undertones of sexuality in a missile dream. Missiles are phallic in shape—if the issue is one of sexual insecurity, then you could have a missile nightmare.

These are some of the most common end-of-the-world themes seen in nightmares. More are possible—the human mind is creative and wonderfully inventive when it comes to thinking up its own destruction. Whatever the particular variation may be, try not to get caught up in the fear evoked by the dream. Step away and try to see it as a message about inner change. Once you gain a sense of objectivity, you can look at your waking life and find the culprit giving you a ringside seat at Armageddon.

# 16

# **P**ROPHETIC DREAMS

There is a long oral tradition of dreams and nightmares coming true. It's often nightmares that are talked of as being prophetic, because the events prophesied are usually unpleasant or even catastrophic. Prophecy has never been a popular profession. It's just too weird, too strange for most to accept at face value. Be that as it may, there seem to be many genuinely prophetic dreams. If I had to make up a definition for these, it would be a simple one: Prophetic dreams tell a story of the future that becomes reality.

My favorite word for dreams predicting the future is "precognitive." I like this word, because it is more readily accepted than "prophetic" by the rational mind. Precognitive is something that occurs "before thought," i.e., cognition. A typical example of a precognitive dream is a dream about someone dying when we know they are actually ill in waking life. Our dreaming mind can put together bits of information and observation that escape conscious notice. We piece together clues leading to a conclusion of approaching death and have a dream. Our unconscious knows what's coming before rational thinking puts the same information together—hence, it is precognitive.

How this kind of information appears in a dream depends on religious and cultural backgrounds and on something else that will never be defined. Every spiritual teaching throughout human history has described or given examples of prophetic dreams. The Bible has many examples of prophetic visions and dreams, as do the Hindu, Buddhist and Islamic traditions. From ancient Egypt to modern-day spiritual traditions, prophecy through dreams has been honored and studied.

When modern people like you or me have something that looks like a prophetic dream it tends to fall into the nightmare category. Usually it scares the heck out of us, because even if the dream is relatively peaceful in imagery, the message is not one we want to hear.

It's easy to dismiss prophetic dreams with some rational explanation comfortable for the person doing the explaining. For example, dreaming of a plane crash and then seeing it "come true" doesn't automatically mean the dream was prophetic. That's because of the frequency of real-life crashes and the possibility it's just dream language for a personal issue. I think that is usually the case, but it's also true some dreams eerily reflect real events and actions.

I have never personally known anyone who dreamed of a plane crash and had it come true, although I have heard plenty of nightmares featuring planes going down with terrible carnage and bodies strewn everywhere. I do know people who dreamed about car accidents that later happened or were very narrowly avoided. In the cases where the accident was avoided, the dreamer took extra care as a result of the dream.

Sometimes a rational approach to nightmares doesn't have all the answers, because some dreams don't fit the usual parameters we use to understand life. Such is the case with prophetic dreams. Stories of prophetic dreams coming true are anecdotal and can never be verified satisfactorily in a scientific sense. For that matter, neither can the whole concept of taking dreams as meaningful and informative events deserving further study. But what are we to make of this next dream? You decide.

*I dreamed about Dad getting shot to death. Then later on that year he got shot six times and died. Then last year I dreamed about my sister getting in a car accident or overdosing on a drug, and within a month she overdosed on heroin. A couple of months later I dreamed about my other sister getting in a car accident and dying. Within a week she got into a car accident. I'm scared to go to sleep at night because if I dream of people dying, I'm scared they will. I think I am psychic and I don't know what to do.*

This is another dream from my Web site. Do you think the teenage dreamer just made this up? It could be, but somehow I don't think so. Reading between the lines, you get a picture of a child living somewhere dangerous, a place where fathers are shot and killed, drugs are a part of life and bad things happen. I get a very strong feeling about this communication out of cyberspace—I think it's true.

How do you know whether or not your nightmare is truly prophetic? The answer is you can't know, until or unless something happens in real life bearing out the details of the dream. That is the nature of prophecy—it can't be verified until after the fact. Even then, you may simply have been unknowingly putting together pieces of information, seeding the dream. I think it's always best to err on the side of reason when looking at a nightmare that apprears prophetic, and to take the approach that it probably is not.

Many nightmares in this book could be thought of as prophetic, especially dreams of disaster and war. Wars, earthquakes, storms and other catastrophic events are always occurring somewhere and are also very popular nightmare themes. If you dream of a great earthquake destroying your town, chances are it's about an internal upheaval, not an actual disaster.

I have known people who actually moved because they dreamed of a disaster. One woman I know dreamed of the dam breaking in the town where she lived and moved a thousand miles away. Oddly enough, she ended up within the flood plain of another dam! For her the breaking dam in the nightmare signaled the release of pent-up emotional content. She handled it well in the end, but for a while she did confuse the inner with the outer reality.

Here's an example from someone who dreams of plane crashes. You be the judge of whether or not she is having prophetic dreams.

*I have recurring nightmares about plane crashes. Sometimes they are commercial airliners but usually they are single-engines. Usually people are killed. They seem to get more vivid and detailed with every one I have.*

*In the beginning they were only planes and would crash over water or land. Now they are as specific as the company names and the colors, and the last time I saw the people, who were not killed. The kicker is that usually I hear of a plane crash on the news exactly three days later, and it has always corresponded with "land or water," "commercial or private." The only one that has not been real is one I had a few weeks ago about a Delta plane going down in a civilian area. I had one about an orange four-seater that went down in the woods behind my house and caused a small fire. Nobody was killed in that one. . . .*

What do you think? Are these prophetic dreams? My feeling is they are not. The three-day time period is interesting, but there are always plane crashes—far more than we usually like to think about. The three-day synchronicity has hooked our dreamer into thinking her nightmares are predicting real events. As she focuses more on the dreams, they become more specific—colors, company names—but there haven't been real crashes bearing out these particular details. She also has at least a fifty-fifty chance of being right about a crash taking place over land or water.

The real giveaway is in the last crash dream she relates, right in back of her house, but with no fatalities and a "small fire." What is crashing is something inside of her, some piece of her life where there is trouble or concern.

If she were to dream of a specific plane, a specific flight number, a company and a crash location that was borne out in real life, then the dreams could be considered prophetic. It's in the details where we can distinguish the difference between a dream that is truly prophetic and one that is not.

Probably the most common kind of nightmare that appears prophetic features the death of someone.

*A little while ago I had a dream that a guy I went to school with and a guy I know got into a car accident. In the dream they went off an embankment and into water of some kind. The guy I went to school with died, because he couldn't get out of the car and drowned. The other guy got out of the car and was all right.*

*Then in real life, a week or so later, I heard from some friends that the two guys did get into an accident—the one I went to school with died and the other one was OK. They had gone over an embankment into some water. Everything happened just the way I dreamed it. Recently I dreamed another guy I know overdosed on drugs and died. Right after that dream, I heard he had really done that and was dead. . . .*

Prophetic? I think so, don't you? These nightmares meet the criteria—they have specific events with specific details seen to occur in real life as they were dreamed.

*My grandmother had terminal cancer and was given thirty days to live. Two days before her thirty days were up, she had a nightmare. She said in her dream she was swinging in a child's swing. She started to fall backward, and she knew that as she fell she was dying, and that when she hit the ground she would be dead. . . .*

This could be seen as a prophetic nightmare, but I think it falls into a different category, one we haven't talked about in this book so far. When people are terminally ill, they often have dreams or nightmares signaling the approaching end of life. Those dreams can be very frightening, or they can bring peace of mind and acceptance.

When you stop and think about it, it makes a lot of sense that we could have dreams or nightmares of this kind. Given that we have nightmares about other things that bother us or create stress, why wouldn't we have dreams reflecting a sense of our own approaching death? Not a popular subject, I know, but that doesn't change the reality. Very sick people will often have a dream of the completion of their life and will tell the dream to anyone who will listen. It can be seen as a blessing or a curse—it depends on the attitude of the dreamer and the one who hears the dream.

If you are in the unfortunate position of caring for someone who is terminally ill, listen to what they say about their dreams. Sometimes medication or other complications of illness shut down the memory of dreams. But if clarity remains, then the imminent end of life will often be signaled by a powerful dream, remembered and told. It is a way for the inner self to let everyone know the time has come. Don't discount such a dream if you are privileged to hear it. Our desire to deny the passing of a loved one can make us insensitive. The relating of a true dream of completion is part of acceptance for the dying dreamer and is a privileged sharing for anyone who can hear and understand it. The dream prepares everyone for completion—that is a priceless gift.

*The night of my grandma's death, my sister had a dream. My grandma was telling her that she was happy now and that everything was going to be all right. My sister was hugging my grandma in the dream.*

This is a different kind of death dream, one that holds out the balm of peace and acceptance. It doesn't matter if the dream was "prophetic," in the sense that Grandma actually died the night of the dream. What matters is the sense of happiness and completion, a genuine solace to the dreamer.

## IF YOU HAVE A NIGHTMARE YOU FEEL IS PROPHETIC

Here's how to approach a nightmare you feel is prophetic.

**Don't panic.** This might sound silly, but people have been known to get very upset when they have a nightmare of catastrophe or disaster. Don't live in fear your dream may come true. For example, you might live in a place where tornadoes are a possibility, but dreaming of a tornado does not mean one is coming in waking life.

**Assume your nightmare is probably not about real events.**
I say this because most nightmares are not prophetic, no matter
how real they may seem to you. Notice I said probably—because
there is always the exception. What I want to get across is the idea
that caution and circumspection are needed if you think a nightmare might come true.

**Make a realistic evaluation of your current life situation.**
Are you under a lot of stress? Is your life situation less than favor-
able? Are there real, external factors that could symbolically appear
in your dream? Examples would include illness, abusive relationships, significant financial stress, or any other high-stress factor.

**Do events in real life closely follow the details in your
nightmare or dream?** If your answer is yes, then you may be
tapping into prophetic areas. If not, then it's very unlikely your
nightmare is about real events. Reread the examples in this chapter to get a sense of the difference.

**Does your nightmare contain any special "markers" to sig-
nal that it is different from your usual dreaming experience?** Genuine prophetic dreams are imbued with a quality missing in garden-variety nightmares. For example, colors may be
extremely vivid, or there is a kind of unique and unfamiliar feeling quality to the dream. There will be something different in a
nightmare or dream that is genuinely prophetic. That fits—if it is
a true prophetic dream, then it must be coming from a very different place than usual. That difference will be reflected in some
way in the dream.

**Does your family have a history of prophetic dreaming?**
Don't laugh. There are lots of people who tell stories about
Auntie's strange dreams or how Great-Grandpa always knew
when someone close to him was in trouble. To this day we still do
not understand what produces prophetic dreams. Perhaps there is
some genetic tendency to break into psychic and prophetic areas

of dreaming, and the gift has been passed to you. However, you still need to look with caution and skepticism at any dream you think might be prophetic.

**Was the information given to you in the nightmare already known to you?** An example of this would be dreaming of the death of someone who is known to be very ill. If the person dies there is no prophecy involved, because it's likely your mind simply put together the logical conclusion death was near, based on information and clues picked up subconsciously (you wouldn't necessarily notice them on a conscious level) and then incorporated into a dream. Since death is frightening to most of us, such a dream can easily appear in nightmare form.

If your dreams are prophetic, try not to let them upset you. That's easy to say, but I know you might have trouble with it, because prophecy is often about unpleasant things. It seems we don't have much use for prophecy that predicts pleasant outcomes and success. Perhaps that's because we don't need to be warned about good things in our lives. It's the unexpected disaster we need protection from, if protection is to come. With prophecy, forewarned is forearmed.

If a dying loved one has a dream of passing, treat it with honor and compassion. See it as a signal transition is near and make your peace with it. It can give you precious time to make good-byes and help you brace for the inevitable.

We don't fully understand why some dreams and nightmares come true, but come true they sometimes do. Use common sense and apply several grains of salt if you or someone you know has such a dream. If it does come true, then try to see it as a sign of the mystery embracing all of us and as a reminder we humans don't necessarily understand as much as we think we do. It's good to be reminded of that every once in a while.

# 17

# OTHER COMMON NIGHTMARE THEMES

If you haven't come across the particular kind of nightmare you are having in the previous chapters, perhaps you will find it here. I could easily write a book about nightmares with thirty or forty chapters or more, but I think my publisher might be unhappy with such a long book—and so might you. I've tried to be as specific as possible about how to look at any nightmare and make some sense out of it. In this chapter you will find several themes not covered elsewhere that turn up with some frequency in nightmares. Remember, the theme of a nightmare provides a clue as to the meaning. All of the following nightmare themes are common, some more so than others.

## *Trapped*

*I walk through a gate. . . . It's one of those creepy metal gates. It leads me to a long stone pathway with moss and things of that sort growing on it. There's nothing on either side of it. . . . As I begin to walk out on it, it begins to collapse, falling into nothing (like a bottomless pit). As I turn and run to the gate, I notice it's closed and locked and I can't get out.*

Lots of things can make us feel trapped in life. Work, finances, relationships, sickness, problems with acknowledgment or love—any and all of these and more could lead to a nightmare of being trapped. Like all nightmares, we must look to the details in order to get a clearer picture of what is upsetting us.

In this case, the dreamer is dealing with some foundational life issues. Anytime you see old, mossy buildings, stones, pathways or steps in a dream, you know you are looking at something fundamental, important and probably unfamiliar to you. These images indicate something old and basic. They refer to areas of the unconscious mind neither brightly lit nor well-mapped. You're on your own when these symbols appear. This dream is very disturbing and it's easy to see why. He's trapped behind the gate and in danger of falling into a bottomless pit, indicating he has little choice in dealing with whatever the collapsing path represents. I would say that something he has relied on in the past is falling apart and is no longer able to sustain and support him. That brings up fear, represented by the bottomless pit. The dream suggests he had better figure out what is going wrong and look in new directions for solutions.

If you have a nightmare of being trapped (or buried alive, or locked in a vault, or otherwise helplessly confined) look to your outer life for some situation contributing to making you feel this way. You may have been denying it or shrugging it off. Your dream tells you it's time to make some changes, even if it's difficult to see how that can be done.

## *Killed*

We are killed in many different kinds of nightmares. There is no end to the creativity of the dreaming mind when it comes to nightmare mayhem. Probably the most common method is shooting, but stabbing, suffocation, being hacked to pieces, run over by a car, wiped out by a bomb, bitten by a poisonous snake or insect, or attacked by wild animals are all popular.

Fortunately for us, we may die in our worst dreams but are resurrected with the morning light. Often a dream may continue after we are killed and we find ourselves in a dream world where life and death have no relationship to outer reality.

*I dreamed I was at my church trying to cook food, with nothing to start a fire but a stick and a stone. I was looking at myself standing in a room, when suddenly someone shot me through the doorway. I watched my head explode all over the wall, my brains and everything. Then I woke up and fell back asleep and dreamed I was walking around with my head all in pieces and blood gushing down my body. Then I woke to my alarm clock.*

The key to understanding this dream is in the setting and in the nature of the wound. Getting shot in the head is referring to something mental, a way the dreamer perceives or thinks about things. The setting tells us a lot. Trying to cook food in a church refers to trying to get spiritual nourishment. But that is not possible for this dreamer—he's only got a stick and a stone to make fire, and that won't cut it. I'd say his nightmare is addressing a spiritual crisis. Perhaps his church is not giving him what he needs in a spiritual sense. Seen from this point of view, the dream is trying to tell him he needs to seek elsewhere for his spiritual nourishment (food). It's saying he needs to get out of the mental and into the feeling and experiential. That is the only way to really get in touch with spiritual realities anyway—our minds can only take us so far.

*My friends and I were walking across the road from our local shopping center, when a car pulled up and a man hopped out. I tried my hardest to run as fast as I could but I wasn't getting anywhere. My two best friends walked ahead of me as the man caught up with me and hacked at my legs with an axe. . . .*

This is another dream of feeling disempowered and helpless. Someone cuts the legs out from under her; it's a phrase we've all heard and used. It also has the classic nightmare feeling of being unable to run or get away no matter how hard you try. Have you ever had a nightmare like that? When you can't get away and your legs feel stuck or impossibly heavy as you try to run, it's a sign you are feeling stuck and helpless about something, unable to get the solution you need. As always, by looking at the circumstances of your waking life, you can probably come up with a good idea about the nature of the problem. Once you know what it is, you can take action to deal with it.

> *In the past four nights I dreamt twice that I was in a big house with a bunch of other people. I guess we were all hostages. There is a gunman shooting at people running around and trying to get away. I am running, too, and end up getting shot. . . . I am under a great deal of financial stress right now and stress at work, but aside from that, nothing else major is going on in my life.*

Here's a quick test of what you've learned about nightmares so far—what do you suppose may be causing this man's bad dreams? Everyone who answered "Stress!" please give yourself ten points. Like most people, this dreamer doesn't seem to think stress is very unusual or could be the reason he's having his nightmare. Nothing else "major" is going on in his life, so why should he be having the dreams? That's his thinking, but he has already pinpointed the cause. Financial stress, workplace stress, either one is enough to get him into a nightmare where he is held hostage and shot. "Held hostage" is dream-speak for a situation out of control. That sounds a lot like his stressful life.

## Someone's at the Door/in the House

I've seen many nightmares where the dreamer realizes something evil is outside trying to get in. Worse, danger may already be inside, even in the bedroom. It can be really frightening, creating instant panic and feelings of vulnerability and defenselessness. It's always been true that the predators among us have never bothered with the conventions most of us live by. In today's world that seems even more apparent. Every day we are bombarded by pictures and stories of the most horrendous human crimes and actions, often involving irrational and murderous attacks on people who were simply going about their business. The stuff of nightmares is all around us, providing plenty of material for our dreaming minds to use in dreams.

It's a challenge in every sense of the word to maintain an attitude of love, helpfulness and trust in waking life. One solution to nightmares is finding an inner sense of self-worth, self-trust and self-appreciation. However it is achieved, nothing drives nightmares away more effectively than this simple truth.

Dreaming of an evil stranger standing at the foot of your bed can be utterly chilling. For most of us the bedroom is a safe and private space, a bastion and retreat against the cares of the outer world. We are at our most vulnerable when we sleep. When we dream of waking to find evil about to attack, panic is the instinctive reaction. If you experience nightmares like this, ask yourself what might be causing a sense of fear and insecurity in your life. It may not be a specific thing; more and more people are experiencing a very broad sense of anxiety about life, for no particular reason they can identify. We can feel frustrated and afraid because we live in a society and world that often appears frightening and dangerous. If you are one of these people, you could easily have nightmares about strangers trying to break in or appearing in your house and bedroom.

The solution is simple, but sometimes not easy to accomplish. We need to connect to others in ways that reaffirm the decent human values of love and mutual support. We need to defuse our fear of others. Some people find comfort in religious community—church, synagogue or mosque. Some find comfort in community activity—volunteer work or community service of some kind. These kinds of activities renew a sense that all is not as the media might have us believe. Although there is much that goes wrong in the world, there is also much that goes right, and there is nothing like a sense of communal belonging and spirit to relieve thoughts of isolation and vulnerability to attack. Try it, you may find that your nightmares of strangers disappear.

## *Nightmare Weddings*

No, I'm not talking about problems with the caterer or pleasing both sides of the family with the arrangements. I'll leave those plots to Hollywood and real life. I'm talking about nightmares— when the ceremony turns into something straight out of hell.

*I dreamed that I got married to a friend of mine, Mike. We were at the church and got married, then went to this enormous building for the reception. There was a massive queue for toilets, which were outside. . . . Apparently people were arguing, so my mother told me to go up there and "smooth some ruffled feathers."*

*I took Mike with me and we walked up there . . . everyone was fine, so we went for a walk. . . . We were away from everyone else when a witch came up behind us (flying on a broomstick) and threw cutlery on the ground in front of us. The witch disappeared, and I picked up the cutlery and we walked back to the hall. But the hall was on fire and there were people screaming everywhere.*

*Suddenly I was running along the veranda beside the hall, and the roof was on fire. There were holes in the floor and people were falling through the holes. People were dying in front of me and I had no idea where Mike was, or my family. . . .*

If that isn't a reception from hell, I don't know what is. I suppose there are some folks who wish the guests at their wedding had fallen into holes, but that's another story. There are usually three main variations in wedding nightmares. One is the disastrous wedding, like the dream above. The second involves everything going wrong and the bride or groom turning out to be some kind of monster or demon. The third involves the beloved becoming horrible and deformed.

To get a sense of what wedding nightmares mean, we need to think about the whole idea of what a wedding is supposed to be. The bottom line is union—union between you (the dreamer) and someone or something else. Unlike sexual dreams, which also have union as an underlying theme, wedding dreams are about making the symbolic union formal and official. When the union turns into a nightmare, you are dealing with an inner conflict centering on some intimate aspect of your waking life. I don't mean sexual intimacy, although that could be a factor. I mean being involved with something in a way just like being married to it. The trick is to exactly identify the source of conflict. There are so many possibilities it's impossible to list them all. You need to play Sherlock Holmes and apply your reason to the problem.

For example, the "marriage" symbolized in a nightmare could be to an idea or concept, especially about yourself. Negative ideas about self fall into this category and can appear in a wedding nightmare as a demon lover, especially if you are actively challenging those ideas in some fashion. Another good candidate is work- and job-related stress. We even talk about people who are married to their jobs—those folks are good candidates for a dream reception in hell.

Perhaps you have been seriously involved with something or someone for a period of time and it's going bad. It could be work or relationship, a career plan, a financial problem emerging—anything significant in your life. You could have a wedding nightmare displaying the ruin of the "union" you have been pursuing. The dream above comes from a young woman trying to come to terms with a growing sense of vulnerability in her world. Cutlery is a classic wedding gift and is also a symbol of nourishment, because we eat with cutlery. When the witch throws it on the ground, it's a gesture of disdain and contempt. Some witch-like aspect is spoiling things. Could it be the mother? I'd look in her direction as a real-life source of conflict and stress. She's the authoritative voice in the dream demanding that ruffled feathers be smoothed.

If you have a wedding nightmare, seek out the source of distress in your life that seems intimately joined to you in some way. Perhaps it isn't something you are already doing but something you are thinking about doing. Are you thinking of "getting married" to something? I don't mean your real-life lover (although it's possible you could have a nightmare about real-life wedding plans) but something else you are considering bringing into your life. You could be experiencing a lot of anxiety about some contemplated change in your life and that anxiety can show up as a wedding horror show.

## *Falling*

Falling dreams are very common and many of them are nightmares. Everything seems so real in a dream that a dream of falling from a high place is as close to the real thing as any of us would ever want to get. There are as many variations as dreamers, but they usually end with a long fall toward certain destruction. Sometimes the ground falls away, sometimes we jump out of windows, sometimes we are pushed from the top of a tall cliff or skyscraper, sometimes we fall out of airplanes. It's always a long way down.

I think falling dreams are mostly telling us we are feeling vulnerable or insecure because of some event or situation. The ground we stand on, the foundation of who we think we are, is threatened or under attack. Here's an example from a woman having a difficult time coping with the loss of an expected child.

*The other night I dreamt I was at the bottom of a high-rise apartment building, and I got into the elevator to go to the thirty-fifth floor. The doors open into an unfinished apartment and there is a big piece of window missing. I tell myself not to go toward the window because I will fall, but something pulls me there and I tumble out. I only feel myself begin to fall, when presto! I'm at the beginning of the dream again and go into the elevator up to the thirty-fifth floor.*

*The dream just keeps going on and on and on! I must have had the dream one hundred times! The only thing that changes in the dream is my awareness that I will fall if I go to the window, and every time I try harder to resist the pull. I fail every time, except the last time the dream happens . . . The last time, I get out of the elevator, see the window and run back to the elevator, which had started to go down again. I jump in the elevator shaft after it, but I never land. . . .*

This dreamer had recently lost her unborn child in the sixth month of her pregnancy. A tragedy like this wounds the psyche, leaving a sense of loss and self-blame. The elevator opens on the unfinished apartment, a dream symbol for the incomplete pregnancy. She is irresistibly drawn out of the window, again and again, because she has not yet resolved the loss. Something is stuck in her psyche, unable to complete. There's good news in the dream, though. It says that even though she is struggling, she will ultimately succeed. That's because she finally avoids the window and jumps after the elevator as it is going down, away from the empty apartment. She has managed to begin a reversal of the emotional damage. If going up in the elevator represents a journey to the place symbolizing the incomplete pregnancy, jumping after the elevator as it starts down signals the beginning of healing and a turning away from the painful emotional trauma. The outcome will be good.

When you dream of falling, ask yourself what is making you feel insecure. It might be obvious, as it is in the case of the woman above. It might not be so obvious, but there will be something you can identify nonetheless.

Falling dreams can also occur during serious illness, like cancer. That does not mean you have cancer if you have a falling dream! I'm talking about people who have already been diagnosed with a life-threatening illness. If you think about it, falling makes us feel completely helpless. Many people who are very ill feel exactly that way. If you are in this situation, my best advice to you is to regain a sense of being in charge. Take charge of your treatment in an appropriate way, asking the questions you need to ask, exploring options and making choices and generally taking responsibility for the way you fight the disease. Don't give up your power to the doctors. Talk with your physicians to establish the right course for you, and resist any attempts to pigeonhole you into some standard treatment box. Get the information you need and act upon it.

If you are experiencing nightmares unlike any of the themes presented in this book, you can apply the ideas and suggestions given throughout and make sense of your particular dream.

# PART THREE

---

# Living with Nightmares

# 18

---

# HEALTH NIGHTMARES

Peace of mind goes out the window when we dream of awful disease. The biggest worry is getting cancer. There are really two kinds of health nightmares. One kind presents images of disease and illness directly, but there may or may not be an actual illness. The other kind of health dream refers symbolically to disease that exists or is potentially present and ready to begin.

I have seen many dreams over the years indicating disease before it appeared and was diagnosed. I have also seen many dreams giving progress reports on diagnosed illness and indicating recovery or death.

The whole idea of dreams that indicated disease and reporting on the success or failure of treatment is very controversial and not broadly accepted. Most doctors would dismiss the idea or ridicule it, since there is absolutely no scientific proof such dreams occur. You can choose to believe what you wish—I can only share my observations and experience. In my experience, dreams are powerful indicators of disease, either of actual illness or as symbolic portrayals of underlying problems. It makes sense that if dreams are a useful way to monitor and understand other aspects of our lives they would also have meaning regarding our health. Health nightmares indicate a crisis of some sort is at hand.

*I keep having this awful dream. I feel my arms turn numb, and when I look at them the veins are standing out about three inches above my arms. I have this dream every night, and each time I wake up rubbing my hands and arms. Could this have something to do with my health? I read in a dream book that it meant something about sorrows and troubles that would never end. It is totally terrifying and even vividly painful in the dream.*

Here's the old dream book again, and this time the reader is doomed to a lifetime of trouble and sorrow. Please don't believe any of those silly interpretations promising doom, misery and loss. There is more than enough to worry about in real life without adding the burden of someone's black fantasies about dreams to the load. How would you feel if someone interpreted your dream to mean you were now set for a lifetime of trouble?

It's awful to see something happen to your body in a dream. Imagine your veins standing out three inches above your arms! We have an innate sense of self, centered on an image of wholeness and good health, a yardstick we use to measure ourselves to know whether we are well or at risk. Veins popping out so unnaturally in real life would be cause for alarm, and they have certainly alarmed our dreamer.

She's having the dream every night; you know by now this indicates urgency. Whatever the problem, it's important. But why veins? Veins are about the circulation of blood. Blood is essential for life, and we talked about some possible meanings for blood in an earlier chapter. They included life, passion and vitality.

Our instinctive response when we have a nightmare indicating something wrong with our body is to take it literally and worry about our health, even if we don't set much store in the meaning of dreams. I would say, in general, that it's always a good idea to get a thorough checkup when such a dream occurs, especially if it

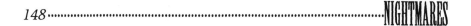

repeats. This particular dream could indicate the presence of circulatory problems, heart disease, etc. A doctor's visit would confirm or deny the suspicion and would alleviate doubt. The dream could also be referring to emotional difficulties. Perhaps things are very blocked and stuck in her life. Blockage in the veins would make them stand out, would symbolically equal emotional conflict—the feelings are unable to "circulate." In any case, a doctor's visit would help clear things up by confirming or eliminating the presence of actual illness.

I recall one woman some years ago who had terminal cancer. Her dreams gave clear signs she was about to die, but at first I did not correctly interpret them. I lost my objectivity, because I became emotionally invested in wanting her to survive. The cancer was represented by trash and garbage littered about in her dreams. Then she had a dream where the trash was neatly bagged and stacked, ready to be taken away. That looked hopeful to me, and there were other things in the dream that seemed to indicate survival. But I was wrong—the collection of the trash was actually a sign she was getting ready to go. She was "cleaning things up" in preparation for her transition.

Another person I worked with dreamed of a cavernous dark lake opening up in her backyard. From out of the lake sprang black, ferocious, prehistoric fish—the kind that seem to be all mouth and teeth. They ate a cat in front of her. Then the dream changed, and she found herself in a room with her mother. There were two annoying teenage girls singing in the room. Her mother said, "I wasn't singing. Don't you know we have cancer?"

A nightmare like this demands a medical checkup. When you get the idea in a dream that you have cancer or when a dream figure says you have cancer, you need to get the checkup just for your peace of mind if nothing else. Some possible dream images of cancer include sharks, prehistoric or monstrous fish (as in this example), tornadoes, excessive garbage and trash strewn about, snakes or devouring insects. That does not mean all dreams including these symbols are cancer dreams! We have already seen several nightmares like this not directly related to a physical problem.

The woman who had this dream was in the midst of a difficult period in her life. She was dealing with upsetting issues reflecting an abusive childhood and adolescence. My feeling about the dream is that it meets the criteria for getting a checkup. It's the kind of dream that could be a precursor to cancer, a warning of what might come. It is also certain the nightmare is speaking about inner emotional issues.

The cavernous, dark lake revealed when the pond disappears is a metaphor for unconscious layers coming to the surface, perhaps a result of her therapy sessions. When the depth is revealed, she doesn't much like what she sees and the dream turns frightening.

Her mother says in the dream that "we" have cancer. This could be dream-talk commenting on the poisonous role the mother has played in this dreamer's life. The fish may represent actual cancer; they may also represent the threatening nature of the issues she is uncovering and confronting in her therapy sessions. Even if the fish do not represent an actual cancer presence, they certainly could represent it in potential.

This brings up a controversial area in medicine: the exact role of the mind in disease and illness. Most physicians balk at the idea of disease directly resulting from psychological causes, unless it's mental illness we're talking about. After twenty years of working with people in various stages of illness, I am convinced there is a direct correlation between mind and body and that the mind can create an unhappy and diseased body. By the same token, we can use our mind to help reverse disease and create a healthy body.

Recognition of the importance of the mind-body interface in medicine is growing, but it's early yet. Some physicians, like Dr. Andrew Weil or Dr. Bernard Siegel, are willing to stake their reputations and their livelihood on exploring the mysterious connection between mind and body. These two well-known authors have helped thousands learn techniques utilizing the power of the mind to promote better health. Their books are available and worth reading, especially if you are seeking information to complement medical treatment you may be receiving.

If it is true nightmares can indicate the presence or the potential of serious illness, then it makes sense to try and understand them. Nightmares can provide early warning or indicate the need for more aggressive action against illness.

*I'm looking at the power supply for my amplifier. It's one of the really powerful old-style tube types, big and heavy. The power supply is smoking and sparking. I see a small flame starting in the middle of the tubes. I'm afraid it's going to burn up or explode.*

When I heard this dream, my first thought was that it was a health dream. Electronic devices (like power supplies, amplifiers, stereos, computers and televisions) are excellent symbols for all sorts of neurological and body activities. If one turns up in a nightmare and it's breaking down and smoking, take notice.

In fact, this man had recently been diagnosed with prostate problems—he told me this after I interpreted the dream with him. It wasn't cancer, but a series of annoying infections unresponsive to treatment. Of course we all know prostate problems make men particularly vulnerable, since there is a potential for impotence and other nasty effects if surgery or other aggressive treatment is required. Seen in that context, a power supply makes a good image for fundamental expression of masculinity. In his dream the unit is igniting and smoking. Not a good dream.

In this instance the dreamer explored several treatment modalities and was able to stabilize the infection. At the same time he has been looking at other nightmares that indicated he must do something to change his work life and find ways to express himself. His creative expression has been stifled over the last fifteen years. A power supply also makes a good symbol for overall self-expression.

I don't think it's a coincidence the infection improved when he took notice of what his dreams were trying to tell him. In effect he got the message and began to do something about it, obviating the need for the symptoms to continue. If he fails to carry through and take action to change things, I predict the prostate problems will return, in a more advanced or dangerous stage of development.

You can see from the above that I firmly believe in the useful-
ness of dreams as valid indicators regarding the state of our health.
It is tricky, I admit, to determine whether or not a dream is just
trying to point out inner conflicts and frustrations or is pointing a
finger at real illness and disease. That's why I always recommend
seeing a physician if in doubt. That's the only way to be sure. Even
if nothing unusual turns up you're only out of pocket for the
exam. You probably needed one anyway, right? And you can't put
a price on the peace of mind that results.

Here's another example of a dream warranting an exam. It also
reflects a common concern in health nightmares—the fear of lung
cancer.

*In my dream I am in a home that doesn't look familiar to me but
seemed like home. I'm not sure why I had to have tests done, but the tests
revealed that I had lung cancer and only a short time to live. I don't smoke
now, but used to. It has been almost two years since I quit.*

*Some of the people in the dream looked familiar to me, some did not. I
told some of the people in the house, but I didn't want my family to know.
I didn't want to tell my daughter or my brothers and sisters. I kept thinking it must be a mistake. I did end up telling my oldest sister, who immediately took charge. She wanted no one smoking in my home. She called
the doctor to get my pathology reports. When I woke, my sister was thinking they had confused my results with someone else's, but I never knew the
outcome because I woke up.*

*I was very upset in the dream. I remember holding on to my husband
and crying. I wasn't afraid to die; I just didn't want to die. I kept thinking, "What would my daughter do without me?"*

If I had this dream, the first thing I'd do is schedule an appoint-
ment for a chest X ray. But I am also inclined to think the nightmare is more about an inner mental state than her health. That's
because I know there was a lot of stress in her life when she had
the dream. At the time of the nightmare her elderly mother-in-
law had just moved into her small house, requiring that the
dreamer and her husband sleep on the living-room floor. That set

up a lot of stress. It wouldn't be unusual to have a dream of getting very ill in a situation like that. It's as if life as she knows it has
ended, even if the situation is only temporary.

Why would her dreaming mind pick lung cancer? She's a
recent ex-smoker, and we have all heard the horror stories about
smoking and cancer. There is a relentless push in our country to
demonize smoking and eliminate it entirely. I see smokers who
want to quit all the time in my hypnotherapy practice. Smokers
often feel guilty and worry that they are killing themselves,
although that is usually not enough motivation to quit. After they
quit, they are concerned for years after with the possible effects of
the past.

We have been conditioned by public policy to equate smoking
with death. If we needed a symbol suggesting suffocation and
death to an ex-smoker, could we find a more chilling image than
lung cancer? In this case, the nightmare could as easily refer to
feeling trapped and suffocated by the changed living conditions as
it could to the actual disease. Only a medical exam will resolve the
question.

Without getting very far into psychology, we all have thoughts
and concerns that can trouble us if they break into our conscious
awareness. For example, if we have negative ideas about ourselves or a negative self-image, those concerns can show up symbolically as a diseased body in dreams and nightmares. A negative
idea might be something like, "I'm not worthy of love," or, "I
cause people pain just by my presence." We learn dumb ideas like
that in childhood, and they seriously affect our happiness.
Sometimes I think the best use of therapy is to help people change
these utterly erroneous ideas about themselves. Here's a dream
that seems to me to reflect this kind of unconscious thinking.

*I constantly have dreams where I have some sort of disgusting rash all
over my body. In the dream it doesn't seem to bother me or other people
around me. . . . It makes me sick and very disturbed to think about it. I
would like to know why I keep dreaming this.*

None of us are really comfortable around someone who has a serious skin disorder or rash. It disturbs us. We tell ourselves it's not contagious; we know it doesn't really matter, but our inner sense of wholeness is deeply affected. We tend to avoid someone who is unfortunate enough to have some disfiguring rash or injury. Our skin is visible to all, and anything that goes wrong with it can be seen by all. It is a very important part of our appearance in the world and a key factor in self-esteem. Just ask any teenager with acne how important it is.

The person who has this dream is uncomfortable with the images. She doesn't like to think about it, and neither would you or I. It's a nightmare about fundamental issues of self-image and self-esteem. Any series of events affecting perception of our self-worth in the world could stimulate a nightmare about diseased skin if we have low self-esteem. Anything that makes us feel outcast, different, unloved, unwanted or incompetent could be behind it. A lot depends on other factors as well, chiefly our overall state of mind and our sense of self as valuable and lovable. This dream calls for reassessment of self from a more positive viewpoint.

If you have a nightmare suggesting health problems, please put your mind at ease and get a medical checkup. My experience tells me most dreams mentioning cancer or some other illness are using the disease as a symbolic image to get something across to the waking mind. Most of these nightmares do not indicate illness. But there are some that do indeed indicate a real, physical problem. Make sure, one way or the other.

# 19

---

# NIGHTMARES AND POST TRAUMATIC STRESS DISORDER

Post Traumatic Stress Disorder, or PTSD, is an increasingly frequent diagnosis among mental-health-care professionals. It wasn't always that way. For years symptoms of PTSD (including dramatic and horrifying nightmares) were either dismissed entirely or attributed to other causes. PTSD has always been around, although it was known by other names, usually related to war, like "shell shock" or "combat fatigue."

PTSD occurs as the result of unacceptable traumatic events in a person's life. The list of possible qualifying events is long, including childhood abuse (sexual, psychological or physical), war-time experiences, violent crime, job-related stress (police, firefighters, EMT people and anyone else with life-and-death responsibilities and experience), accidents, and terrorism (like the Oklahoma City bombing). In fact any significantly traumatic experience involving actual or potential serious injury or death, or which otherwise terrifies the victim in some fundamental way, can qualify as a possible cause.

Sometimes it's not necessary for the person suffering from PTSD to actually be in direct danger. Confrontation with violent death can be enough. Witnessing a terrible car accident or a murder could lay the foundation for PTSD. The more severe the trauma, the more intense the symptoms.

It's no fun living with PTSD. The person affected does not sleep well, which leads to a constant state of sleep deprivation, irritability, poor co-ordination and lowered energy. Often the person doesn't know what's wrong—why things bother him (or her) so much, or why he keeps jumping on people who are only trying to love and support him. There is a real tendency to feel threatened and paranoid, a sneaking suspicion things will turn bad at any moment. As if that isn't enough, all this is accompanied by nightmares—recurring, ongoing, horrific dreams that wake the sufferer in a cold sweat, yelling and thrashing, perhaps striking out at the person lying next to him.

Treatment focuses on medication and therapy, but is frequently complicated and limited by the unwillingness of insurers to cover the costs of effective long-term therapy. Many people never get very far in the therapeutic sense and come to rely on drugs to suppress the symptoms. There is also a tendency in our society, still very strong, to dismiss therapy as a symptom of weakness. Police, military personnel, firefighters and other people in traditionally dangerous professions look with suspicion on the idea of talking with someone about traumatic events occurring in the course of their jobs. Moreover, outsiders are not fully trusted, since they are not part of the profession in question. That limits many to in-house psychologists, who may be perceived as a threat to career advancement. No one wants a visit to a psychologist on his job record. This attitude is changing as more people recognize that PTSD is a normal response by our psyche to levels of stress produced by the real threat of serious harm or death.

Nightmares and waking flashbacks are characteristic of PTSD. Often the dreamer relives the traumatic events in dreams, either exactly as they occurred or with variations playing out the underlying theme of mortal danger. In flashbacks the person is awake but gets caught in a waking nightmare, reliving traumatic events as if they were occurring in present time.

I don't know of any easy way to deal with PTSD nightmares. The only thing that really helps folks who have PTSD is compassionate and competent counseling, coupled with loving support from friends, relatives and family. All the drugs in the world won't do it—the inner mind needs to consider the issues and repair the damage done by the traumatic event. That requires skilled and patient guidance. Peer groups of trauma survivors can help a lot, because shared experience and retelling of the events can go far towards defusing the charge.

There is great reluctance on the part of some people with PTSD to talk about their experiences with counselors who are not peer-group members. That is especially true with war veterans and paramilitary organizations like the police. I understand their concerns, because the lack of shared experience can make for a genuine barrier to understanding. Theoretical approaches alone won't cut it with PTSD. Even so, there are many qualified therapists with direct experience of danger and coming into harm's way. That can establish the common ground and mutual respect that is critical, in my opinion, to therapeutic success. If you are a person with PTSD, please don't limit yourself to peer-group members for help. Ask around—you will likely find someone in your community who understands.

PTSD nightmares will diminish or even disappear with successful therapy. What seems to make the difference is whether or not the sufferer is able to find a new sense of safety and security in life. It is like rebuilding oneself from within, finding something in the rubble of the devastated psyche that can be used to create a new foundation of self.

I'm not going to give examples of PTSD nightmares here. The nature of the particular trauma will be reflected in the dreams. Vets relive combat, police dream of car stops turning deadly, firefighters are trapped in the flames—whatever the nature of the stress, it will be reflected somehow in the nightmare scenes.

How do you know if you are suffering from PTSD? You can't

know for sure unless you are diagnosed by a professional, but there are a few general criteria that point in this direction. These are red flags to a therapist, and perhaps they may resonate for you. If you or someone you know meets these criteria, you should seek a professional opinion. Self-diagnosis is always risky, so take this list as simply a starting point. Some of these, like sleep problems, can easily indicate something entirely different and may have nothing to do with PTSD at all.

## SOME COMMON INDICATORS/FACTORS IN PTSD

- Traumatic and repetitive nightmares.
- Sleep problems: insomnia, fitful sleep, night sweats, fatigue and exhaustion.
- A life history that includes very traumatic events: accidents, war, childhood abuse, violent crime, domestic abuse, work-related events, anything that brings up a confrontation with complete helplessness and personal mortality. This is the most important criterion.
- Depression and a feeling life is meaningless.
- Self-esteem problems related to the traumatic event(s). For example, rape victims frequently experience severe self-esteem problems.
- Excessive feelings of guilt related to the traumatic events (survivor guilt).
- Dysfunctional behavior—doing things that interfere with going about the daily business of life (drinking too much, taking drugs, skipping work, inability to hold a job or work regularly at something, abusive behavior towards loved ones, etc.).
- Deep-seated frustration at not being able to "just get through it."
- Repeated flashbacks or vivid memories of the traumatic event(s) that will not go away.
- Difficulty controlling emotions—anger, grief, etc.
- Thoughts of suicide.

These are some of the common criteria and factors associated with PTSD; many are also associated with severe depression. The key indicator, of course, is the history of traumatic events. Sometimes it is a cumulative effect, as is often the case with police officers and emergency medical personnel. Years of exposure to danger and to the uglier side of human activity takes its toll.

All of the ideas throughout this book for looking at nightmares can be useful if you are suffering from PTSD and are trying to understand your dreams. But in a way, you already know why you are having them, don't you? The unconscious gets stuck on the bad events and tries to resolve the psychic wounding through dreams. It's like a sore tooth—the dreams keep probing at the sore, trying to soothe it and bring relief. I can offer a few, basic tips that may help you get past it.

## WHAT TO DO IF YOU THINK YOU HAVE PTSD

**Seek professional help.** I know this may be old news to you, but if you haven't talked with someone you owe it to yourself and to those who care for you. It's a complex problem that requires guidance.

**Find a way to tell your story, as many times as you can, to as many people as will listen.** The more you tell it, the more possibility of reducing the "charge." Find someone who genuinely listens—you know the difference between someone who is polite and someone who is genuinely present with you.

**Trust your intuition about whom to work with in a professional sense.** Ask some hard questions: What is that person's experience of life? What is the common ground? Look for real-life experience and appreciation of mortal danger.

**Recognize this truth: it is entirely normal and appropriate to have the kinds of stressful reactions you are experiencing.** Yes, normal, because no one except a fictional movie hero escapes emotional scarring from traumatic events. Once you really understand that your response is normal, you have stepped onto the road to recovery.

**Be patient—it takes time to rebuild the inner sense of self that has been traumatized.** Rome wasn't built in a day and neither were you.

One technique for handling difficult nightmares is discussed in chapter 22—lucid (conscious) dreaming. It's not for everyone, but it might at least give you a handle on the dreams and help you find a way to come to terms with the source events. It won't always apply and you will still need guidance to get through all the twists and turns of PTSD. But it can help.

One last thought—if you have PTSD you can get through it and come out on the other side. You can find the peace of mind you are looking for. You are not alone, and there are many that stand ready to help you. All you need do is seek them out.

# 20

## WHEN CHILDREN HAVE NIGHTMARES

Few things produce feelings of helplessness for a caring parent like the sobbing of a terrified child waking from a nightmare. Anyone who has been around young children knows the reasons for an upset are usually not understood by children, and often not by the parents themselves. A nightmare is an upset, horribly real to the child and important enough for the parents to address. When your child starts crying, it's not a good time to brush the whole thing off as "just a dream."

Nightmares are very common in children, typically beginning at around age three. They may continue, on and off, through ages seven and eight or beyond. Can you put yourself in your child's shoes? A child is not in charge of things. The world is at once fascinating and threatening, full of rules and booby traps at every turn. Very large people called adults are always directing you to do or not do something. Everything seems much bigger than you are. Much of the time people don't understand what you are thinking or trying to communicate. You are dependent on others for love, food, caring and safety. Any one of these may be in short supply, and all bets are off once you enter school and leave the familiarity of the home to engage the outside world on your own, a place where bullies lurk and not everyone is nice to you. In the best of circumstances, children will still have nightmares as they attempt to integrate and make sense of the enormous and complex world around them.

You can make it a little easier for your child by taking positive steps to help him or her integrate and come to terms with the bad dream. The first step is realizing a child's dream ought to be taken seriously—you need to pay attention. Paying attention is a conscious act of parenting that pays off in happier children and a better relationship between child and parent.

## Listening to the Dream

Children don't really care much about what the scary thing in their dream really means. You may know the dream monster chasing your kid at night has something to do with the stress of a family situation or an external factor like starting school, but the child doesn't know that. All the child knows is that when he or she goes to sleep, a horrible monster appears. The first task is to actually listen to the dream without trying to help the child "figure it out" or dismissing the dream as unimportant. If you ignore your child's feelings you may do long-lasting damage to your relationship.

## Getting Control of the Dream

The best solution to nightmares is to eliminate the underlying cause of distress. That isn't always easy or possible, even if you have a good idea about what the underlying cause really is! The next best thing is to help your child gain control over the dream, so it no longer frightens or returns. But how do you do that with something as elusive as a dream?

The answer is to be creative and present. By "present," I mean fully focused on your child and not wishing you were back in bed or that you could hurry things up somehow. The time to defuse a nightmare is on the spot. It might mean taking time to engage in conversation about the dream and then doing something creative and proactive to give your child a sense of power over the frightening images. It's only a few small minutes lost from your sleep but it's a very large measure of support for your child.

For example, after letting the child know you realize how scary the dream is, you could mention that everyone has these dreams sometimes. You could say you used to have scary dreams, but you figured out how to make them go away or how to scare the monsters away so they wouldn't come back. You could get out some paper and crayons and help draw the dream—this can be very effective. Then, after drawing the scary image, perhaps draw something to show that your child is stronger and bigger than the nightmare monster, or has special "powers" (like the Power Rangers on television) that makes the monster retreat. You get the idea. Use your best judgment about how far to take this in the middle of the night, but be sure to follow up the next day.

By the way, it's perfectly OK to tell your child to attack and fight the monsters and kick them out of the dreams. In today's politically correct culture, there is a growing tendency to label as bad anything that appears in any way violent. Punching a monster is certainly "violent," but it is also important for the child to feel there is some avenue of action to follow. You can also tell your kid to yell at the monster to go away. Whether or not your child actually does these things in a dream is not important; what's important is the idea there are real options to confront and defeat the scary nightmares.

Role-playing can be very effective. Sit down with your child the next day and create a plan for dealing with the monster or scary thing. Let your child make suggestions. Perhaps the monster can be locked up in a box, or Batman can be called to come scare it away. My grandson likes Batman and the Power Rangers, so these are very powerful symbols to him of super-hero strength and support. These fictional characters are real to him at this stage of his life, so in his mind it's logical they could rescue him if things got scary. He learned he could kick the monster out of his dream.

Once you've created the plan, play out the story. Pretend to be the monster and then retreat in terror as the super friends are summoned. Call for help once you are locked in the box or whatever has been decided. Make yourself "disappear," like the wicked witch in *The Wizard of Oz* ("I'm melting . . ."). By turning the nightmare situation into a game where your child wins, you teach the conquering of fear.

All of the things causing nightmares in adults cause nightmares in children as well. Too much stress, illness and fever, medications, peer pressure—these are just a few of the common villains. It's up to you, as the parent, to try to minimize as many of these factors as possible. You can make the effort to keep it easygoing at home and find ways to let your child know he or she is loved and safe.

## THINGS THAT HELP CHILDREN WITH NIGHTMARES

Here's a brief list of things you can do if your child is having nightmares.

• Let your child know the dream is important to you and that you really know how scary it was.
• Encourage your child to tell the dream several times. This helps defuse the feeling and "energy" of the dream.
• Ask your child to draw the dream and then talk about the drawing. You can use this as an entry into developing a plan to deal with the nightmare.
• Devise a plan together to make your child feel there is a way to deal with the dream.
• Role-play the plan and go through it a few times to anchor the idea in your child's mind.
• Encourage and reassure your child, especially at bedtime. Fear of having the dream again may very well come up as bedtime approaches. If necessary, play out the plan again.
• Identify causes of stress in your child's environment and try to eliminate or modify them.

The last item needs a little discussion. Unless your child is ill, chances are the nightmares are a result of various stressful events. Some are difficult to address. For example, just going to school and learning to be away from home is difficult for a kid. Since the situation is inherently stressful, the best thing you can do is to try to soften the impact with reassurance, love and awareness. By awareness, I mean paying attention to the school environment, communicating frequently with teachers or caregivers, and in general taking an active and involved role in the educational process.

If things are tough at home, do the best you can. Whatever is upsetting you, it's your stuff, not your child's, and it's important not to dump it on the kids when things get to be too much. The payoff is less stress = happier children = a more peaceful home environment all around.

Remember, nightmares are normal during child development. The best response is acknowledgment, love and active support to re-establish a sense of security.

## *Night Terrors*

Night terrors are different from nightmares. The difference can be seen in the behavior of the child. Though nightmares may cause a child to wake crying or screaming, night terrors are much more dramatic. A child having night terrors will violently toss about and loudly cry out during sleep and can be very difficult to wake. Sometimes bed-wetting can accompany night terrors. The dream is usually not remembered.

Night terrors generally occur in the first two hours of sleep. No one really understands what causes night terrors, and there isn't a specific cure for it. It does seem to be stress-related. Night terrors may continue for some time, but usually will go away on their own. If they are persistent and long-standing, you may want to consult your physician.

The good news is that there really are things you can do to make a difference if your child has nightmares or night terrors. Please give the ideas contained in this chapter a try. You have nothing to lose except, perhaps, a little sleep and a little time. The reward can be sleeping peacefully and contentedly through the night for both you and your child.

# 21

## TEEN NIGHTMARES

Teenagers have it rough. They're not old enough to have full freedom and command of their lives, nor young enough to be forgiven mistakes in the same way they were as children. A confusing and often dangerous society confronts their ability to learn and grow safely. Mechanistic educational policies, temptations that would please Satan himself, and physical and emotional changes that can't be ignored set them up like no other group for nightmares.

My wife and I ran a teen nightmare survey on our Web site for teens from thirteen to twenty years of age. The survey was anonymous, with no way to reply or ask for further information unless the participant provided an E-mail address. We asked a lot of questions, ranging from age and sleeping habits to the frequency and kind of nightmares the participants were experiencing. We received almost 700 responses. The frequency of different kinds of nightmare themes changed, to a degree, in different age groups, but overall showed a lot of consistency and carried through all ages. Twenty-one percent of these teen dreamers had nightmares once a week or more! That's a lot of nightmares. Fourteen percent of teens responding had them every two weeks, fifteen percent every month and twenty percent every three months. If this sampling is any indication, there are millions of teen nightmares happening on any given night.

Teenagers have different concerns than adults and those concerns show up in their worst dreams. Issues of relationship, peer acceptance, coping with school and work, leaving home, parents and other authorities, danger and accident all figure prominently in their nightmares. Though breaking up with your boyfriend may seem relatively unimportant from an adult point of view, to a teenager it can be dramatically upsetting. If you are a parent of teens, you know exactly what I mean. It's no surprise nightmares about breaking up are common.

Chase dreams are the number-one nightmare theme among teenagers. Fifty percent of the teens responding had awful dreams of being chased. The next most popular theme was accidents. One thing comes through in the comments from different teens: The dreams are very frightening to them. They don't know what to do with them, what they mean or how to handle them.

The comments made on the survey are very revealing. They say a lot about how teens struggle with their developing role in the world and about their concerns, symbolized by everything from monsters to unknown killers chasing them. Sometimes the comments reveal sleep disorders that need medical intervention, sometimes they tell a tragic story of childhood gone terribly wrong.

If you are the parent of a teen, the kinds of frightening dreams your children reveal (if they will trust you not to dismiss them!) will tell you a lot about what's going on with them. You don't have to be a psychologist to see that the themes of your teen's nightmares can honestly reflect their real problems. The dreams will present mini-dramas about the things in life important to them.

It's perfectly normal for teenagers to have nightmares. It's not so normal if they are having nightmares every night. High frequency of nightmares can be a sign of being overwhelmed and of

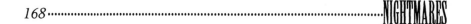

excessive stress. It's up to you to discover the causes. Aside from the normal stress of having to do all the things teens are expected to do, perhaps there is some situation that adds to the burden, creating fertile ground for nightmares. Can you change something to lessen the load? Are you contributing to the stress, perhaps with unrealistic expectations or well-meaning indifference? Here is a small sample of the things teens say about their nightmares and how they feel about them. They reflect a broad spectrum of concern and life experience.

## Failure

*At least twice a week I have nightmares about failure. Failing to do well in school, failing to get a part in a certain play, failing to master my major, failing in life in general."*

This comment from a seventeen-year-old girl is typical of many we received. Fear of failure ranks high as a stress factor for many adults—how much more so for teens, who are not yet empowered to set their own boundaries and standards for success?

## Sleepwalking

*I sleepwalk and talk sometimes during them and feel embarrassed when I hear about it from my mother the next day. I'm afraid I'll hurt someone. I've hurt myself several times before.*

This thirteen-year-old dreamer has REM sleep disorder—sleepwalking. It will probably clear up, but could signal an ongoing problem. Her nightmares are about being chased, being wrong, her house burning down and seeing accidents happen. Her parents need to get a doctor's advice, because sleepwalking can be dangerous to everyone concerned, especially the dreamer.

Accidents are the second most common theme in teen nightmares, according to our survey. Usually the dreamer sees someone close and loved, friends or family, being injured or killed.

## Accidents

*There are a lot of times I am just watching someone get hurt or in danger and I am completely unable to help them."*

*I have nightmares all the time about my dad falling asleep at the wheel of a car with me in the passenger seat, and he hits and kills a lady in the street. The lady looks right into my eyes as she is hit. Every time I close my eyes I see her.*

*I usually dream about people close to me having an accident.*

Often teenage dreamers are worried their dreams about accidents will come true. In every case they dream of the loss of someone loved or close to them, or that they are helpless to prevent some tragic event. Such dreams speak to the fear of loss, the idea that in an uncertain world things and people we love can be taken from us without our permission.

## Being Chased

*I'm always hiding from killers. I'm always being chased, close friends or family are usually being chased with me as well."*

*My nightmares are usually about being chased and hunted by something supernatural.*

*Most of my nightmares are reoccurring ones about being chased by lions, cheetahs, etc.*

*They really scare me. They are always so realistic that I sometimes don't know if it really happened or if it was a nightmare.*

*At least once a month I get nightmares so violent that I'm nearly falling out of bed and my sheets are either tangled around me or on the floor. I wake up sweating, breathing hard and crying. The dream feels so real that I find myself watching behind my back the rest of the day.*

The last two comments exemplify another common response: The dreams seem so real they affect waking life and reality. Does it help to point out that dreams aren't real? What do you think? Try telling that to a teen who is frightened out of her wits by a nightmare. It's better to simply acknowledge the fear and then gently try to find out what lies behind it.

Being chased in a dream means exactly what it seems to mean: Something is chasing the dreamer—not in the sense of people or attackers but in the sense of life pressures building and making the dreamer feel driven and harassed. Since teenage life is crammed to the brim with life pressures, it makes sense that being chased turns out to be the most popular nightmare theme. The way to deal with chase nightmares is to find a way to reduce the pressure.

## Can't Breathe

*Once, in real life, I started coughing and couldn't breathe for a while and my face turned blue. It was traumatic and happened one other time. From time to time I wake up in the middle of the night and the same thing is happening. But after a few seconds I calm down. It is very frightening.*

Medical problems of any kind can produce vivid and frightening nightmares. The boy who has this nightmare gets it at least once a month. He dreams of suffocation and accidents. He could be suffering from apnea, a sleep disorder that affects breathing. Apnea can be life-threatening, cutting off breath and placing enormous strain on the heart and respiratory system. Whatever the problem is, his dreams emphasize the need for a medical opinion.

## Demons and Violence

*Everything is extremely violent and horrific. I've never seen such horrific scenes in my whole life. Even my imagination couldn't come up with the stuff that is in my dreams.*

This young woman dreams of demonically possessed animals trying to kill her. Her dreaming mind presents images to her seemingly beyond her waking mind's imagination. But nothing is impossible for the unconscious, including the unimaginable and horrific. The animals in her dreams may represent an inner struggle with primal and unknown forces of sexuality awakening within her; they may represent a real threat from her waking life.

## Nightmares Rooted in Physical and Sexual Abuse

One of the most pervasive real-world threats to teenagers is an abusive parent, perhaps combined with living in a dangerous environment or home situation. Unfortunately this is a common nightmare theme for teens. Abuse by a parent or other adult is common and under-reported. The next several comments and nightmares reflect the reality of adults abusing the children who should be under their protection.

*I keep dreaming about things that happened with my stepdad, being abused—*

*I can't tell the difference between dream and reality anymore.* [This dreamer was physically abused.]

*When I was seven my father died. In my dream a ball of light is chasing me. I always fall just stepping out of my room. In my mind I am asleep but awake. My father used to beat us.*

This last comment comes from a teen having nightmares every night since she was seven. Even though her father is no longer there to beat her, he's still after her in her dreams. You could say that what is after her is her sense of insecurity, her lack of safety and her history of abuse. The ball of light is an example of how our dreaming mind can conceal the actual nature of what is troubling us. Perhaps it's easier for a seven-year-old (now a teenager) to deal with an anonymous ball of light than an image of her own father chasing and attacking her. She also dreams of running away from home and of people who are mean to her. Are you surprised?

*I have nightmares about normal or silly stuff that shouldn't even be scary. But for some reason I'll be so frightened that I wake up, and then*

*I'm so freaked I can't go back to sleep. Sometimes it's just the overall mood or tone of the dream that's scary. I also have the same nightmares I had when I was little—like slimy, slithery things that sting in my underwear and lions in the hallway between my room and my mom's, or being trapped in a cage.*

*I was sexually abused when I was little and I have the same dreams I had when I was little, and it was happening. I'm depressed often.*

These are classic nightmares. It doesn't take a genius to make the connection between slimy, stinging, slithery things in her underwear and the sexual abuse. That is even more apparent because the dreams are the same ones she had as a young child. The lion in the hallway symbolizes inability to reach the protection of her mother—she can't get to where her mother is, and her mother didn't protect her in real life. I am constantly amazed and saddened in my practice by the amount of childhood abuse that the people who come to me have experienced. Child abuse is devastating, often making it almost impossible for the adult to feel normal and happy. This young woman would certainly benefit from therapy to help her get through the issues appearing in these dreams. She also dreams of spiders, appearing undressed and vulnerable, sex, being chased and people who are mean to her. Do you begin to see how nightmares mirror inner emotional struggles? Teenager or adult, it's the same story.

It's possible to use nightmares as a key for understanding, opening the door to healing and renewal.

*My father is an abusive man. I didn't realize this fully until I began having vivid dreams almost two years ago. These were mostly dreams about being chased. My father was symbolized by darkness or unknown danger, once as a tiger. I give these dreams a lot of credit for getting me out of my relationship with him. I had a dream last night that I think might be about him, where I was chased by a black cat. The cat was set on hurting me and seemed to get out of any trap I set for it—which, unfortunately, is how I feel about my father.*

Here's a disturbing dream, all the more so because of what is left unsaid by the boy who shared it. He's fifteen years old.

## Sex

*I've been having the same nightmare almost every night for eight years. The only differences are in small details and the people (because I move very often, and when I do the new people I meet take the place of the old). In the most frequent one I am trying to escape from some place or some uncomfortable situation. It usually ends up with me dying. The point where I die is the most disturbing, because when I die in a dream it doesn't end. I either go to hell or I just sit in the coffin after the funeral looking at my tomb, unable to move.*

*The dreams were OK at first. I just didn't care about anything, because I had a really horrible childhood. But then I moved out from my dad (the cause of most of the trouble), and my life got better but my dreams didn't. Recently they have been getting worse. Now they all involve me dying. They all involve some kind of monster (god, Satan, mythical creature, people with super-human powers) trying to catch me and kill me, as well as me and three or four girls acting in many sexual escapades that I wish I could have with them. (But they all die too.) There's something new: the addition of drug addiction in my dreams. In all of them I am strung out on heroin or crack or something like that (which is why I always get caught—I'm always too high to move very fast).*

I wonder where this boy lives and how he's doing? In his dream world Satan chases him down, killing him and the symbols of his budding sexuality and inner desires as well—the girls in the dream. Sex is a common teen theme in nightmares. Wouldn't you expect that? It's hard enough as an adult to deal with the complex emotions and events of expressing sexuality. It's much more difficult for a teenager.

The addition of drugs in his dream is ominous—is he now taking drugs? I can't ask him, so I don't know. Our dreaming mind will use any image from our environment or experience to make a point. Drugs can be seen as a metaphor for a kind of false power to alter unpleasant reality. Taking drugs is an expression of the unconscious psyche, both in dreams and in real life. If he is really taking drugs in waking life, the dream is warning him of a dangerous potential. If he is not, they are a symbol of everything that is going wrong for him, holding him back and making him vulnerable.

*I always have dreams that I'm captured by some male figure, and I will try to have him release me by seducing him or even flashing him. The sexual nature of this dream is disturbing to me.*

Here's another sexual dream, from a seventeen-year-old girl who dreams of snakes and secret rooms. Often teens (and adults) are disturbed by the raw sexuality presented in nightmares and other dreams. Usually someone is uncomfortable because the dream actions don't agree with their waking thoughts about what is OK and what is not. It's normal to have dreams and nightmares about sex. I could write many pages about sexuality in dreams. It helps to remind yourself that sexual acts in dreams do not mean you are actually seeking to express the images in real life. Sexuality in dreams means much more than just some suppressed desire or fantasy.

In the dream above, sex becomes a way to protect the dreamer from the male who has captured her. She offers herself, hoping to escape. It's a tactic employed countless times throughout history by women who found themselves at the mercy of male captors. It's a last-ditch attempt, based on a need to survive at any cost. Something is really troubling this dreamer and she needs to discover what it is. She's a teenager trying to cope with becoming an adult. It may be a dream about emerging sexuality; it may refer to a threat or a situation in real life.

## Bad Relationships

*I keep having dreams that my boyfriend kills me and leaves with someone else, or that something happens to him and he's taken away from me.*

This is a common theme in teen nightmares. Teens easily become attached, discovering the drama of involvement with someone, exploring the meaning of love and affection. Many teens fear the loss of love. It's a natural theme for teen nightmares.

Since the Columbine school shooting in Colorado and the widespread media coverage that followed, more and more teens dream of violence at school. Often they worry a shooting will happen at their school—that it's going to happen to them. It's another example of how we pick up on events in the larger world and incorporate them into our nightmares. It's the randomness and unpredictability that scares us. For a teen attending high school it would be hard to find a better symbol then Columbine for feeling vulnerable. That is the everyday experience for most teenagers.

Teenagers aren't stupid—if they can figure out a way to handle the dreams, they will. They may also discover a connection between their waking lives and the source of their nightmares. Here are two relevant comments from the survey that reveal a very good understanding.

## Consciously Working with Dreams

*I usually have nightmares if I go to bed angry or upset about something and I have not resolved it before going to sleep. I think that is what triggers my nightmares.*

*For a lot of my life, up to when I was thirteen, I had horrific nightmares almost every night. It was only one day when I had a kind of lucid dream that I was able to conquer my fear and realize I could put an end to my nightly horror. I just wanted to mention that it really changed my life and it may help other people as well, who knows?*

Lucid dreaming is a technique for controlling the dreaming experience. That could come in very handy if you are having a series of awful nightmares. I don't know what caused the years of nightmares for the second dreamer, but she's spontaneously discovered a tool for exploring dreams that is subject to a lot of research and study. Lucid dreaming techniques are discussed in chapter 22. It's possible to change nightmares and master the terror they create.

The first dreamer has nightmares of being choked. That's a good symbol for feeling "choked" by anger and frustration. She has made the connection. Maybe she's headed for a career in psychology! Going to bed angry and disturbed sets the stage for nightmares and disturbing dreams. It's a significant realization to put the two together.

What can you do if your teenage son or daughter is having frequent nightmares? The key here is the word frequent. A nightmare once in a while is perfectly normal. Frequent nightmares indicate a more serious degree of upset and stress and you need to do something about it. If you are a teenager reading this chapter, the things I recommend here are things you can do to help yourself.

## HOW TO HELP WITH TEEN NIGHTMARES

**Make an effort to listen.** This is probably number one in all categories of teenage life, so why not with nightmares as well? One of the biggest problems is miscommunication between parents and teens. It doesn't take much to know that, does it? Yet parents frequently tend to forget it. Too often a parent's idea of communication means telling the teen something. Real communication is a two-way street and requires effort on the part of both parties. So please, don't brush off your teen's nightmare as "just a dream." It's important to talk about it.

**Respect the feelings revealed in the dream.** One thing about nightmares is they always involve feelings—embarrassment, shame, guilt, anger and more. No one's going to tell you anything unless they get respect for the way they feel. It doesn't take much to turn off trust in this area. Perhaps you can recall times when parents or others simply ran right over your feelings, without a clue they were doing so. Don't make the same mistake. Nightmares leave teenagers feeling vulnerable and frightened, and it's a good idea to stay sensitive when you are listening or trying to help.

**Know when you are out of your depth.** By this I mean it's possible you need professional help if your teen is experiencing repetitive nightmares. It's one thing to talk about a bad dream now and then; it's another when those dreams are happening all the time. You are not supposed to know how to handle difficult dreams, nor to know what they mean. What you need to know is that such dreams may signal real distress, and you owe it to your child and yourself to find out what's causing it and then do what you can to alleviate it. This book may help, but some circumstances go beyond the capability of any self-help book to resolve the issues.

**Help your teenager maintain a sense of balance in life.** Balance is something we all have trouble maintaining from time to time. By balance I mean a healthy division between work, play, activity, sleep, learning (school) and just plain relaxing. I know it's impossible to get it perfect, but do your best. I also know it can be a struggle, so you have to weigh the benefits against the downside of attempting to regulate your teenager's life. You have to do it, but you need to strike your own balance, based on your best judgment, of when to push and when to back off.

**Be aware of unusual sleep circumstances.** If other things are also happening when your teen is asleep, like sleepwalking or gasping periodically for breath, think about seeing your doctor. You could be dealing with a sleep disorder, which is treatable. Sleep disorders are very common, but are not well publicized in our society. A sleep disorder can rob your teen of happiness, success in school and psychic well-being. Anything that severely disrupts sleep has to be handled. Teens don't do well without sleep and neither does anyone else.

**Make sure your teenager gets enough sleep.** Sleep is critical— most teenagers need up to ten hours of sleep, and most do not get it. In our survey we found a direct correlation between feelings of unhappiness and depression and a lack of sleep. Modern sleep research backs up our findings, proving that lack of sleep will make it very difficult for your teen to function well in school or at any other activity.

I would be hailed as a genius if I could provide easy solutions for the things that stress teens out and give them nightmares. I don't have those solutions, but the next best thing may be for you to take the time to listen and respond when your teenager comes to you with a disturbing dream. You may not be able to "fix" whatever is disturbing things; it may just be part of growing up and coming to terms with the larger, adult world. Some things cannot be altered, and teenage disappointments and frustrations are a part of life. But at least you can keep the lines of communication open and show your teen you care.

# 22

WHAT TO DO WHEN YOU WAKE

Taking the fear out of nightmares requires knowledge of whatever is bothering you so much that a nightmare is needed to make you take notice. We dread the unknown, but the familiar is at least something we can understand and respond to as needed. The best strategy for dealing with nightmares is to make the unknown known and make an effort to understand the meaning of the dream. Just making the effort may be enough in itself.

## Conscious Control of Nightmares (Lucid Dreaming)

There is a technique I'd like to share with you if you are frequently troubled by nightmares. It's not my personal favorite, because I believe the best solution lies in understanding what is behind the dream and then doing something about it. For me that offers the most potential for inner growth and relief from difficult dreams. Even so, many people have benefited from learning how to become aware in their dreams and then using their new aware-ness to confront or challenge the nightmare events. This approach is called conscious dreaming or lucid dreaming.

In a lucid dream you become consciously aware you are dreaming. You are still in the dream and the dream activity is still happening but your perspective changes dramatically, because you now know you are dreaming. Since you know it's a dream, you are no longer caught up in thinking everything is real. If a dream monster approaches, or a murderer intent on dismember-ing you, you now know it cannot harm you. You can initiate action in the dream, stopping attackers or beginning a conversa-tion with them to find out why they are causing so much trouble.

This approach is excellent for gaining a sense of power over your nightmares. It may or may not reveal anything about the underlying cause but it does let the dreamer feel a lot better. If nightmares have been driving you up the wall, this might be the tool to use.

How do you do it? The trick is to teach yourself to become aware (while still actually asleep) when you are dreaming. There are two basic approaches you can follow. One method uses a device to flash low-intensity light on your eyelids when you enter a REM (dreaming) state. The light signal acts to trigger your awareness of dreaming without waking you. Once you become aware in the dream you can begin to change the dream events if you wish. These devices may be found and purchased on the Internet.

The second method works well but takes a little patience and practice. In this method you use a body cue to trigger awareness in the dream. One I have used is simple: you trace a letter on the palm of your hand, pushing firmly into your palm and thinking how this letter will remind you that you are dreaming when it appears in a dream. It can be any letter you like. The first letter of your first name, the letter Z because you like Z, C for conscious-ness, or any other letter that speaks to you in some way. Here's the sequence:

## INITIATING CONSCIOUS DREAMING

1. Trace the letter you have chosen ten times on the palm of each hand, using your finger. You can also actually write it on your hand in ink and glance at it from time to time during the day to remind yourself you are learning about conscious dreaming.
2. As you press the letter into your palm, tell yourself this is a cue for conscious dreaming. Tell yourself when you see the letter in your dream it will be a signal to your awareness to become lucid.
3. Do this again before you go to sleep.
4. Do this at odd times during the day, whenever it occurs to you.
5. Write the letter you've chosen down on sticky notes and post them in odd places where you will see the letter from time to time—it's a reminder you are learning how to dream consciously.

That's all there is to it! It does take a strong desire to enter conscious dreaming states, and it may take a week or two, even more, to see results. But if you stick with it, sooner or later you will find yourself awake in the middle of a dream. Then you can decide what you want to do from there. If you would like to find out more about lucid dreaming, check the Internet. Use search words like "lucid" or "conscious dreaming" and you will quickly come upon sites with more detailed discussions of this ancient technique.

## *Conclusion*

I hope you have found the information in this book useful. Use it as a resource; if your particular nightmare doesn't quite fit into any of the themes I've listed, then read through and get a general sense of how to go about discovering the meaning. There is a lot of information here, based on twenty years of practical experience. The suggestions for understanding any particular theme may apply equally well to a different one, or to one that has not been discussed.

Most of the chapters contain very specific ideas and suggestions designed to help you identify and deal with the underlying cause of a particular kind of nightmare. Refer to the chapter focused on the theme of your bad dream and you may find what you need to uncover the cause.

There are only two requirements for successfully working with nightmares. The first is this: Accept the idea you actually do have the ability and information you need to figure out the meaning and get the message. It might take a little effort to ferret it out, but if you do, your reward will be a peaceful night's sleep. The second requirement is harder for many folks: you must be willing to tell the truth to yourself about how you feel. Often a nightmare appears because we have successfully denied our feelings about something unpleasant and emotionally painful. It can be disturbing to face that honestly. Nightmares are not simple things, and they often refer to significant hurts and psychic injuries we have accumulated. That's why it's sometimes necessary to seek out counseling for permanent relief, especially if the dreams are recurring or frequent.

If you don't really want to get into the psychology of it all, I understand. It's not everyone's cup of tea (or coffee, as the case may be). Still, it does require some effort on your part. No one can just hand you the answer, even though that is probably all you really want. Most of us just want to know what the darn thing means and not get into a lot of discussion about it. That's why I've tried to give guidelines all through this book, focusing on the most common problems and themes.

Here's a simple summary, a step-by-step guide to working with any kind of nightmare, regardless of theme, duration or cause. By following these few steps you can effectively begin to take the charge out of your nightmares and perhaps discover why they are happening. Sometimes you may need assistance from someone else, a professional or a friend, to get to the real meaning. But if you follow these steps and refer to other chapters in this book dealing with your particular kind of dream, you can get results. Then there is a very good chance the nightmare will not return.

## *Simple Steps*

**1. CALM DOWN AND DISTANCE YOURSELF FROM THE EMOTIONS OF THE DREAM.**

Most of the time we get so wrapped up in the feeling of a nightmare it takes several minutes to calm down enough to even think about doing something about it. So the first thing to do is just that: calm down, take a few breaths, and realize you are safe and protected in your own bed. Even if you have been dreaming about terrible things in that same bed, it's a nightmare, not reality.

The old trick of telling yourself "it's just a dream" is fine for openers, but if you've read this far you know I don't think that approach is enough. It doesn't deal with the real reason you are having such a horrific dream. What it does do is give you a place to stop and take stock of the dream. It's just a dream, it's true, but you need to make sense of it and act upon it. By reminding ourselves it's a dream we take the first necessary step to understanding: distancing ourselves from the emotional content so we can arrive at an objective perspective. Then we have a chance of getting to the bottom of it. As long as we are caught up in fear, grief, anger or any other emotion triggered by the dream, we will not see it clearly.

**2. REMIND YOURSELF THAT A NIGHTMARE IS JUST A WAY FOR YOUR INNER SELF TO GET YOUR WAKING MIND TO NOTICE THAT THERE'S SOMETHING YOU NEED TO KNOW.**

This is a little bit like number 1, because it helps you distance yourself from the scenes and emotions of the nightmare. What you do is begin to apply reason and your innate ability to understand the meaning to the dream. Something in you brought you the dream, so something in you must understand what it means and why you had it. The wisdom of your inner mind has decided to hit you with your own dramatic horror show, and it's up to you to do your part and figure it out. Think of it as an interesting challenge, a puzzle you can solve, and you will be well on your way to discovering the meaning.

### 3. RECORD THE DREAM AS BEST YOU CAN—DETAILS, COLORS, IMAGES AND EVENTS.

Write it down or narrate it into a tape recorder. You will forget important details if you don't. Then you can look at it at your leisure later on, when the light of day makes it easier to think through the problem. Details fill out the story, just like the sets of a movie or the descriptions in a novel. Sometimes the real meaning of a nightmare is hidden in the details.

### 4. TAKE A LOOK AT YOUR WAKING LIFE AND SEE IF YOU CAN IDENTIFY A PROBLEM AREA.

Work, relationships, traumatic childhood memories and events, family problems, stress, PTSD or illness can all result in nightmares. Are any of these problem areas for you? If you are dreaming about demons in your work cubicle, it might be logical to assume work has something to do with the problem. I know one man who had several awful dreams featuring his briefcase. The briefcase was a metaphor for his career and work situation, in all of its complexity. The meaning of his nightmares was clear: Do something about it or you will be in serious trouble. It was time for him to make a change.

It's harder to pin down more nonspecific images, such as a faceless enemy pursuing you. One thing you can safely assume: stress is a factor in any nightmare. If you can get a handle on the stress, you can get a handle on the dream. Sometimes it's a little more complicated, because you cannot easily point to an obvious source of heavy stress in your current, waking life. If that's the case, see the next suggestion.

### 5. RELAX AND ALLOW IMAGES AND IDEAS TO FREELY ASSOCIATE.

Free association is simply allowing things to come together of their own accord. For example, if your childhood was not good a nightmare image of a childhood home may call up feelings and memories of helplessness and vulnerability, or even trauma. Then you know the dream is trying to get you to deal with these old issues in some new way.

The trick with free association is letting it take you where it may. Ask yourself, what do I think of when I think of the nightmare image? Write down the image and then write down your thoughts about it. For example, suppose you dream of a fire burning down your house. You write down the image, then you list all of the thoughts or ideas you can associate with the image. These might include destruction of your way of life, loss of safety, loss of structure, helplessness and more. While doing this you might get a gut feeling about the meaning. In this example, perhaps the house burning down represents fear over the end of something in your waking life, some framework or structure dissolving. It's the kind of image that could occur if there are serious relationship problems in a marriage, if you lose your job, or if you find yourself in any situation where life is suddenly insecure and in danger of significant change, especially unwanted change. See how it works?

**6. ONCE YOU HAVE AN IDEA OF THE PROBLEM AREA IN YOUR LIFE, THINK ABOUT POSSIBLE WAYS TO IMPROVE THINGS.**

Sounds like a no-brainer, but we all know this isn't always easy. Just the same, give it a shot. There is always something to be done. Ideas about our limitations are often the biggest obstacle preventing us from doing something to positively affect our situation. It doesn't hurt to ask for spiritual guidance if things seem too difficult to solve. I'm serious—it doesn't matter what religious background you have or what particular beliefs you follow. My experience is that even people who don't think of themselves as either religious or as believers in some divine intelligence get help when they ask for it. What have you got to lose?

Make a plan to deal with the problem. Most of the time we can make changes and remove the need for any more nightmares. A plan is essential. Without a plan, nothing happens. It may only be a short list of things needed to improve things. You can develop that into a full-blown plan. Then you must follow your plan to get the results. If it's a serious problem it might take some time to resolve it, but you can do it if you set your mind to it.

Don't be afraid to ask for help if it seems beyond your abilities. There are lots of resources available for just about any situation you can think of. Many communities offer free or low-cost counseling, support for getting through physical and emotional problems, help with parenting, employment opportunities and advice, financial support in one form or another, or spiritual counseling from leaders of local places of worship.

If all this seems a bit much to consider for dealing with a nightmare, then take whatever seems of value to you and leave the rest. Some nightmares don't have much significance and can disappear with something as simple as a good night's sleep. But others reflect serious issues and concerns. If you have one of these, you will intuitively know it. Then perhaps you may benefit from following the steps above.

My purpose in writing this book was to create a practical guide for understanding our darkest and most terrifying dreams. We all have them—it's a common thread in our human experience. Once we get past the roller-coaster fears a nightmare creates, it's possible to tap into a powerful resource of self-healing and well-being. All we have to do is want to do it.

Thanks for coming on this journey with me. May all your dreams be a source of inspiration and knowledge to you.

# APPENDIX

---

*A Glossary of Common Nightmare Symbols
and What They Mean*

Everyone wants a quick fix when it comes to understanding nightmares. I wish it were as simple as that. There are so many ways to look at nightmares it's impossible to accurately pin down the meaning of yours in a general book like this one. What I've put in these pages is a grab bag of different techniques and ideas to help you sort it out. This appendix is one more item in the bag.

The problem with trying to interpret nightmares (and other dreams) lies in understanding the exact nature of the symbols appearing in the dream. Everything in a dream is a symbol, from the floor under your feet (if there is a floor) to the clouds in the sky overhead. Every detail, every item you notice, every color, every sound or sight or action must be considered.

Obviously it's impossible here to make a complete list of nightmare symbols, much less define their meaning. You have your own associations and meanings for anything that is seen in a nightmare. However, it is true many symbols have a more universal meaning and content. It is also true we can make some very broad generalizations about what some of these may mean. We can use those generalizations to start the process of free association leading to understanding.

I dislike dream dictionaries stating a particular symbol means a particular thing, but find myself in the odd position of feeling a list of common symbols will be helpful to those of you who want to understand what your nightmares mean. I ask you to take this glossary for what it is—my attempt to make a list of some common nightmare symbols with suggested possible meanings. It is an incomplete list, because there are so many potential associations for just about everything and because anything can be seen in a menacing and nightmarish context. As an example, you may love flowers, but if flowers appear in the hand of a dream murderer chasing you with an axe, they take on a new and frightening meaning. If flowers aren't on the list but they show up in your dream, then it will be up to you to figure out the association of something you normally do not fear with a nightmarish action or image and discover the meaning.

The list is in alphabetical order, so you can easily glance through it and see if the particular image you are looking for is here. If not, check the index and see if you find something leading to a particular example or discussion elsewhere in the book. For example, in the chapter on blood you may have noticed a detailed list of meanings for wounds to different parts of the body. Throughout the book, symbols are sometimes defined in the context of discussing a nightmare. The index will guide you to them if you don't find them here.

All of the symbols listed below are relatively common in nightmares. There are an infinite number of potential symbols in any dream, because each of us has an infinitely complex life experience. There is plenty of raw life material for our dreaming minds to draw upon. If the images in your nightmare are not found here, you can gain understanding by carefully reading this book and applying the suggestions frequently given for understanding different kinds of nightmares. The underlying principle is always the same. Let your mind freely associate possible meanings for any particular symbol and the chances are good you will get a sense of the meaning.

## COMMON NIGHTMARE SYMBOLS

**911:** This emergency number never responds with help in most nightmares. If you do get an answer on the dream phone, chances are you will be disconnected or told no help is available. In Nightmare Land, 911 is usually a symbol of trying to get assistance. Assistance for what, and from whom? That's a question you will have to ask yourself. See **Phone.**

**Abyss/Pit:** Depending on the dream action, the abyss can represent the depths of the unconscious, a descent into some hellish possibility, or just sheer terror and abandonment. It's dark and bottomless in the abyss, signaling primal fear.

**Accident:** Accidents occur when we lose control, so they are a good symbol for feeling exactly that. You find yourself speeding down a hill with no brakes, or in some other difficulty. It's usually a serious accident in nightmares.

**Airplane:** Planes are usually crashing in nightmares. Because we are not in control of airplanes (unless you are a pilot, in which case the symbol becomes even more powerful), a plane crash can signal confrontation with your inability to prevent or affect something.

**Aliens:** Aliens are totally unfamiliar and in nightmares are threatening. Therefore, you are feeling threatened by something foreign or unknown to you—sometimes not in your conscious awareness. Aliens can pop up when your mind is trying to introduce new and uncomfortable psychic material to your waking awareness.

**Alligators:** Ancient life forms, alligators symbolize primal forces considered dangerous by the waking mind. Primal forces include sexuality, survival, and violence.

**Barrier (wall, fence, etc.):** Just what it looks like—something standing in the way of understanding or that forms a division between one thing and another. A symbol of feeling unable to get to something or through something.

**Black Figures:** Figures representing something not consciously known. For people of dark-skinned descent, a symbol of the deeper unconscious can appear as darker or blacker than the dreamer.

**Black Man/Woman:** In addition to the above, the gender of the figure and the way it appears can tell you something. Old, young, powerful, sick, etc.—all these things will give you a clue. How does the figure act in the dream? The gender may offer a broad clue to follow for understanding. Male figure—look for mental, structured, ordered context. Female figure—look for chaotic, intuitive, non-linear, feeling-level context.

**Blackness:** In general, things that appear black in a nightmare are referring to unconscious thoughts and context. Blackness may symbolize something hidden from conscious appreciation and understanding.

**Blind:** Blindness or seeing a blind figure in a nightmare often refers to "not seeing" something. It could also signal something concealed or hidden, being "blinded" by something.

**Blood:** The essence of life force, fear of mortality and death, fear of pain, vulnerability, helplessness, being drained of life, passion. See the chapter on blood.

**Bodies:** A comment from the unconscious on death and fear of death. Can represent inner, psychic upheaval needing to be addressed.

**Body Parts:** Theme of dismemberment; what is dismembered? See the chapter on blood for more information about specific parts of the body. Almost always some underlying theme of powerlessness and vulnerability.

**Bomb:** Bombs in your dreams represent something "explosive," e.g., unexpressed, powerful emotions. Nuclear bombs (and missiles) represent total destruction or annihilation and a potential for inner change and transformation. Nukes mean something is ending in a big way, or is trying to reach completion in a psychic sense. We are constantly changing on an inner level; sometimes inner growth is preceded by a nuclear nightmare. Anything nuclear is in itself a symbol for something fundamental.

**Buried:** Something "buried" in your unconscious, hidden from your waking mind. It could be something you've repressed (unscientific term—stuffed) or refused to deal with emotionally. Digging something up in a dream means you may be starting to deal with the underlying issue.

**Cape/Cloak:** No longer a common article of clothing, a cape symbolizes covering over something, cloaking it, hiding it in the unconscious. The nightmare figure of Dracula wears a cape because the vampire represents darkness and life-threatening evil, and because his character was created in Victorian times, when capes were common. His cape covers the dark nature of his reality.

**Car:** The nightmare car typically breaks down at a crucial time; sits menacingly, waiting for you to get in; won't let you get out; or goes out of control. Often, there will be some horrible force riding along, or something/someone else is driving. Cars can refer to the physical body or the "vehicle" by which you get things done. A car can symbolize the way you see and do things in life, the way you go about your life, your perceptions. See **Vehicles**.

**Clouds:** In nightmares, usually storm clouds gathering ominously to signal an approaching storm. Clouds can block the light. "Light" can refer to reason, spirit, or just plain understanding.

**Clown:** The clown is a figure of terror for many children, until they realize it's supposed to be funny. Stephen King capitalized on this in his novel *It*. Nightmare clowns are symbols of something hidden behind a false appearance. The nature of the underlying reality is not in accord with the way in which the waking consciousness sees it.

**Coffin:** A fine symbol of change and transformation. Also something buried, hidden. If you find yourself in a coffin, you are undergoing some kind of inner shift. It may take a while for that shift to emerge in outer reality. It may also mean you feel that your life is in a "deadly" place, *i.e.*, unnourishing and pointless or meaningless.

**Crypt/Vault:** A tomb, a place where dead things are left. It's another image of change. Significant change is fearful to us, which is one reason dreams of death and entombment frighten us so much. The crypt becomes a symbol of the context—change and transformation of something within.

**Dead Baby:** If it's your actual child, can symbolize the ending of something that is a part of you. "A part of you" means anything you are doing or manifesting in your life, actions, ideas, etc. If the dead baby is not a real character, then it can refer to something trying to emerge from you (ideas, changes, etc.) that has come to no fruition. A tricky one to understand fully, because you have to identify what it is that has "died."

**Dead/Wounded Pet:** We project many things onto our pets. Losing a pet is like losing part of our family. A dead or wounded pet in a dream usually means emotional loss or disturbance.

**Dead Friends, Relatives, Family Members:** Please see the chapter on this subject. A complex symbol that cannot be easily categorized.

**Death:** Death as a symbol signals transformation, ending, change and potential new beginnings. You have to think it through to discover what is ending or finished. Usually a sign of impending change of some kind.

**Death's Head:** Like the coffin, a symbol of death and therefore change, ending, etc.

**Demon:** Demons symbolize forces of unstoppable and fearsome evil. If they show up in your dream, you are feeling threatened about something and completely helpless about it. A very powerful symbol—dreams with demons need to be looked at to get to the root of things. Please see the chapter on this subject.

**Devil/Satan:** The devil is the biggest demon of all, so he appears for emphasis. Can also reflect religious upbringing, as he is the Father of Lies, the Tempter, etc. Examine the actions of the dream devil for clues as to the meaning. See the chapter on demons.

**Disease/Illness:** Usually not referring to actual health problems, although this is possible. As a symbol it does indicate something is "ill" in the dreamer's psyche. By looking at the dream image you can get a sense of what is meant. For example, skin disease could indicate a problem with self-image and self-esteem. The nature of the dream disease offers insight into the nature of the problem.

**Dismemberment:** Almost always referring to feelings of disempowerment in some area of life. See the chapter on blood for more information. If you are dismembered in a nightmare, something is tearing you apart emotionally. Also, transformation of self.

**Doctor:** A physician may refer to health issues. If he or she is a demonic or dangerous doctor, the image can symbolize fear of authority or fear of finding out something is physically wrong with you. If the image is a negative academic doctor (Ph.D.) then the emphasis shifts to self-criticism and authority issues, perhaps feeling invalidated about something. A positive doctor image in a nightmare is a good sign that things will turn out well in the end, whatever the underlying issue might be.

**Drowning:** Please see the chapter on suffocation. Drowning is a symbol for feeling overwhelmed by something. Could be brought on by complications like asthma or apnea.

**Earthquakes:** Very common image. It can indicate generalized anxiety about things (for example, you live in California and are worried about "the big one," or you worry that life in general is not safe). It can signal an internal or external upheaval in your life or feelings of vulnerability in some life situation.

**Enemies:** Symbolic nightmare images of internalized fears. Can also mean specific people or threats in your life situation.

**Evil Force:** As a non-specific figure, evil is a symbol for the psyche's basic fear about something seen as extremely threatening to one's sense of self. A nightmare of confronting ultimate evil may signal a major change in life or in one's inner growth.

**Falling:** Falling is a common dream event and is not always nightmarish. In a nightmare it can mean you are feeling unsupported or refer to loss of control and a sense of helplessness and vulnerability.

**Fence:** See **Barrier**.

**Fire:** Fire means transformation and change. Fire destroys by consuming the outer form and reducing it to ash. As a nightmare symbol it implies the dreamer is disturbed by change taking place in inner or outer reality.

**Flood:** Like fire, flood destroys, but unlike fire the form or structure is not transformed. Floods are about feeling overwhelmed, usually in an emotional sense. A flood can also refer to powerful spiritual forces stirring in the dreamer's psyche. Like water, a flood as a symbol does not lend itself well to simple definition.

**Fog:** Fog conceals things. Fog is about confusion, not seeing something clearly, getting caught up in some unconscious action. A barrier to clear knowledge about something. In nightmares, whatever comes out of the fog is a key symbol for understanding the underlying psychic disturbance.

**Foreigners:** Like aliens, foreigners are unfamiliar, something foreign to conscious understanding. If you have a nightmare featuring foreigners, then you will need to dig a little deeper to find the meaning.

**Frozen:** If something is frozen, it often refers to something suppressed or denied. By implication, relief may be found through expression and integration of the repressed emotions or feelings.

**Gangsters:** Gangsters are uncontrollable and dangerous. They break the rules. A good symbol for feeling menaced and at risk of something, afraid about something.

**Ghosts:** Lots of children have nightmares about ghosts. To children they symbolize the unknown, fearful things in life. It's not much different for adults. Ghosts are lifeless and unnatural things. They can become dream symbols for feeling unnourished and unloved, or fear of becoming abandoned and alone. In other words, a dream ghost indicates some feeling of disconnection from life and underlying terror about the consequences of that disconnection.

**Glass:** If the glass is clear and can be seen through, like a window, then it can represent an emotional barrier or refer to something rigid and inflexible. If the glass is broken or shattered, then it could symbolize the breaking up of old beliefs, ideas, barriers, or other rigid areas of life. There are many possibilities for this symbol, depending on the way it appears in the dream. It needs to be considered in context. A drinking glass could refer to issues of nourishment.

**Grave:** Another symbol of change and transformation. A death symbol. If you see a grave in your dream, something is either completing or has the potential to complete. Or you could be looking at an image of "burying" something, i.e., stuffing and repressing it.

**Gun:** A classic symbol of attack. The gun is a masculine image because of penetration by bullets, the shape of the weapon, etc. If you feel threatened in some way by a male, men, or masculine ways of doing things, this symbol could appear.

**Hanging:** Could refer to a problem with breath and breathing. It could symbolize something left hanging, i.e., undone or unfinished. Also a frightening symbol of unpleasant death, so it will often refer to some basic insecurity.

**Hospital:** A hospital is supposed to be a place of healing but can symbolize death to many folks. The context indicates an emotional or psychological problem that needs to be "healed." In nightmare hospitals, things may not go well.

**Illness:** See **Disease.**

**Insects:** Please see the chapter on insect nightmares. Insects have many different symbolic meanings, depending on the kind of insect and what it is doing. At the risk of making a bad pun, perhaps something is bugging you.

**Knife:** Like the gun, a knife is a masculine symbol. It's a symbol of fear. A knife can be much more frightening than a gun, because it cuts and opens the skin. A very good symbol in nightmares for vulnerability and mortality.

**Laughter:** In nightmares, nobody's having any fun when laughter rings out. It's usually demonic and evil. Can signal basic feelings of humiliation and helplessness.

**Lesions:** See **Disease.** The location of the lesion offers a clue to the nature of the underlying issue.

**Men Chasing:** Fear of the masculine. This symbol can refer to issues with authority, feeling threatened and out of control, or to a general level of high stress about something in life.

**Money:** Nightmare money refers to issues of nourishment and support.

**Monsters:** Children often dream of monsters, because monsters are an excellent symbol of the unknown and undefined anxiety. Adults dream of monsters when things are really getting out of hand and they feel threatened at fundamental levels. A good example of adult monster nightmares can be seen in the *Alien* movies, starring Sigourney Weaver.

**Mud:** Mud is dirty, slimy; it covers things over. We talk about politicians "slinging mud." Mud as a nightmare symbol can refer to body problems where some form of internal cleansing is required. More frequently, mud symbolizes covering something up or feeling "bogged down" by something.

**Nameless Fear:** Nameless fear is exactly that—a fear not consciously identified. It can be a symbol for generalized anxiety or can signal an internal awareness of something going wrong before the conscious mind has become aware of the problem. It can sometimes be associated with health issues.

**Nazis:** For most people Nazis in nightmares symbolize evil, an implacable, merciless force that cannot be reasoned with. Nazis are a symbol of mental, unbalanced and dehumanizing forces.

When the SS shows up in your dreams, it's time to take stock of your outer life and bring in a nurturing balance. A complex shadow symbol of unconscious and destructive forces we all contain.

**No One Hears Me:** More of an action than a symbol, when no one hears you it's a nightmare comment on how you are feeling inside. Chances are you are feeling somewhat helpless and invalidated.

**Paralyzed:** Just what it seems—you are feeling helpless and stuck about something. Paralysis is an actual physical effect during hypnogogic experiences. If you experience hypnogogic dreams (see index) you are most likely under severe stress. You need to do something about it.

**Phone:** The phone is a symbol of connection to others, communication and access to help (see also 911). Usually there's something wrong with phones in nightmares. If you get a clear connection, try to remember what you hear on the other end of the line. If you can recall what was said, you will have first-hand information from your inner self about the nightmare problem.

**Plague:** A variation on disease, plague is all-inclusive and widespread. In other words, it's a symbol of a very broad-based problem. Something like a bad career situation or a bad marriage of some duration might show up as plague. Probably referring to a problem of long-standing and widespread influence.

**Police:** A symbol of authority. Like every other dream symbol, it has to be considered in context. If you are a police officer it means something very different than it would for someone who is afraid of the police or is a criminal. Often in nightmares the help and assistance represented by the authority of the police is not available. If you are chased by police in your dream there is an authority issue for sure, probably coupled with feelings of victimization and helplessness.

**Radio:** Like the phone, a radio is a symbol of communication. In nightmares information can be given over the dream radio. Pay attention.

**Rape:** A symbol of helplessness, victimization, fear and violation. The dreamer's boundaries are destroyed. Can appear in PTSD dreams, based on real-life events.

**Red:** All colors are symbolic. Red is like blood and can refer to life, passion, anger and blood.

**Satan:** See **Devil**.

**Scorpions:** Another common symbol, like spiders and snakes. Scorpions frighten people—they are primal, poisonous and menacing to most of us. They can sting, even sting themselves to death. A good symbol for self-loathing, issues of self-esteem and self-judgment. Also may refer to concerns about being "stung" about something.

**Sewage:** Sewage in nightmares is a warning about something, either on a body-oriented or feeling level. Something needs to be cleaned up or changed when this symbol appears.

**Sex:** Sex is obviously a very complicated symbol. The bottom line has to do with union with something. In the image of the nightmare sex lies the clue. You are engaged with some inner force or issue, symbolized by the partner or by the sexual activity you are viewing in the dream.

**Sharks:** Sharks are ancient, dangerous and threatening. They can appear if the dreamer is feeling threatened in outer life. They can also symbolize an internal disease, like cancer. Sharks devour: cancer devours from within by destroying healthy body functions. Feeling attacked in your business life? You could dream of circling sharks.

**Skeleton:** Another death symbol; see the death definitions above. Can also refer to something stripped down to essentials—the bare bones. It will signal change of some kind.

**Skin:** When something's wrong with the skin, something's wrong with the outer appearance of things. If it's our skin, then perhaps there's a problem with the way we see or present ourselves. If it's someone else's skin, look for a clue in the nature and quality of the other figure.

**Skull:** See **Death**.

**Snakes:** See the chapter on snakes. Can symbolize sexual issues or may refer to knowledge or wisdom about something. Depending on cultural background, the snake may be associated with evil.

**Snow/Ice:** When something is covered over with snow or ice it is without heat, i.e., it is lifeless and without passion. Usually refers to emotional issues. See also **Frozen**.

**Soldiers:** Another authority symbol and a symbol of an unstoppable force. When armies appear in your nightmares, you are feeling threatened.

**Spiders:** See the chapter about spiders. A common nightmare symbol. Something that entraps you.

**Stairs:** Stairs in nightmares inevitably lead to bad places. Going down stairs can symbolize a fearsome descent into the unconscious. Going up stairs may lead you to some horrific image of inner fears you would rather not deal with.

**Stuck:** Feeling stuck and unable to move or move quickly is a classic nightmare scenario. It's a symbol of helplessness and inertia, a feeling of being unable to escape from whatever is bothering you.

**Suffocation:** Also a classic symbol, it's very much what it appears to be. Something is "suffocating" you, repressing you, holding you back. It may refer to internal or external issues. You can have suffocation dreams with certain illnesses. Please see the chapter on choking and suffocation.

**Suicide:** This image can appear if you are unfortunate enough to have been closely involved with someone who committed suicide. The mind is trying to resolve and understand the event. It may also appear as an inner image of self-rejection or denial.

**Television:** Television sets can symbolize information: not just the information itself, but the whole complex process of how we receive, integrate and express ideas and thoughts. It's a symbol of perception and can present key nightmare material directly in visual scenes on the screen. When you are watching a TV program in your dreams, it's a good idea to try and remember what you see. Television sets and computers may also refer to the brain, if the dream is about a specific health issue.

**Throat/Neck:** The throat or neck usually refers to self-expression in dream language, depending on the dream action. If your throat gets cut in a nightmare (a common event!) you can bet there's a problem with expressing yourself in some critical way. If someone's head gets cut off, then the throat can be a symbol of the connection (or lack of it) between "mental" and "feeling" (head and body) ways of doing things.

**Tidal Waves:** Tidal waves are a frequent image in nightmares. They occur in dreams during times of unsettling emotional stress or when life seems overwhelming. If the wave is seen on the horizon, perhaps you are being alerted to rising levels of stress or psychic discomfort. If the wave is towering above you or sweeping all before it, then you may have already arrived at a place of upheaval, one of those junctures in life where change is unavoidable and unwelcome.

**Toilets:** Toilets are about letting go of something, eliminating something. In health-oriented nightmares they can symbolize the need for internal cleansing or the need to detoxify the body in some way.

**Torture:** Something feels like torture, e.g., a relationship gone bad or some other unpleasant and ongoing life situation. Torture is also a symbol of feeling victimized or helpless about something.

**Vehicles:** Vehicles come in all shapes and sizes. The type of vehicle contains a specific message for the dreamer. For example, there's a big difference between a broken-down brown Chevy and a shiny new red Ferrari. By looking at the color, condition, passengers, dream action and events surrounding the appearance of a nightmare vehicle, you can learn something about the underlying meaning of the dream. Vehicles can represent the way in which we do things (how we "get there") or they can symbolize the body.

**Wall:** See **Barrier**.

**Watching Loved Ones Die:** One of the most upsetting nightmare symbols. Generally refers to feelings of helplessness or fear of being alone.

**Water:** Water is a universal dream symbol and can take on a wide variety of meanings. The kind of water, the color, the depth, the condition (*e.g.*, turbulent or calm) and more affects the meaning. For example, a dream ocean may refer to the unconscious mind or to spirit, to the feminine psychic principle, to emotional issues or to something completely different. It's not possible to give a simple interpretation for this symbol. It helps to see the water in your dream as a metaphor for something in your life. Like vehicles, the many possible appearances of water must be looked at through the lens of personal experience to reach understanding.

**Wild Animals:** Wild animals cannot be controlled, so one meaning is feeling helpless and at the mercy of something. Wildness is dangerous; the dreamer feels threatened by something. Wild animals are also instinctual and undomesticated, so another meaning is that the dreamer is trying to deal with primal and instinctual feelings and psychic urges. "Psychic," in this sense, refers to the unconscious and essential content of our minds.

**Window:** A window can be seen through, but it is a barrier also. It serves to separate us from something. Windows are brittle and rigid. These qualities will have something to do with the underlying meaning of the nightmare.

**Witches:** Witches have been around for a long time as a symbol of evil, destructive, dangerous feminine forces. Society has always feared the unleashed power of women, and the witch has symbolically taken on all of the negative thoughts about women existing through the centuries. Children frequently dream of witches chasing them—it's a common childhood nightmare. When adults dream of witches it is generally referring to negative ideas and experience of women and the feminine. The witch can represent a distortion of feminine values and purpose, or can refer to feeling threatened by an external situation.

**Women Chasing:** Many nightmares feature men chasing the dreamer with dark intent. When women are chasing you, the meaning is different. It could be the dreamer has an unpleasant history with women. It could also symbolize a problem in balancing "masculine" areas of life (structure, work, mental approaches, etc.) and "feminine" areas (intuition, spiritual areas, chaotic elements, etc.). The meaning depends on the dreamer's ideas about the roles and nature of men and women and on his or her life experience.

**Wolves:** Wolves have become a collective symbol in our society. To the rancher protecting his livestock they are dangerous preda-

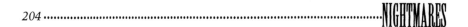

tors; to the conservationist they represent freedom and a return to balance in the environment. What do you think about them? In any event, they are undomesticated and therefore represent a force not easily controlled. Whether that seems dangerous or not depends on your viewpoint, but if you are attacked in your nightmare, you can safely assume you need to seek out the real-world cause of your alarm.

# INDEX